THE LADY'S HANDBOOK
FOR HER
MYSTERIOUS ILLNESS

THE LADY'S HANDBOOK
FOR HER
MYSTERIOUS ILLNESS

Sarah Ramey

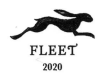

FLEET

2020

FLEET

First published in the United States in 2020 by Doubleday,
a division of Penguin Random House LLC
First published in Great Britain in 2020 by Fleet

1 3 5 7 9 10 8 6 4 2

Copyright © 2020 by Sarah Ramey

The moral right of the author has been asserted.

A CIP catalogue record for this book
is available from the British Library.

HARDBACK ISBN 978-0-7088-9885-7
TRADE PAPERBACK ISBN 978-1-8440-8724-2

Printed and bound in Great Britain by
Clays Ltd, Elcograf S.p.A.

Papers used by Fleet are from well-managed forests
and other responsible sources.

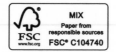

Fleet
An imprint of
Little, Brown Book Group
Carmelite House
50 Victoria Embankment
London EC4Y 0DZ

An Hachette UK Company
www.hachette.co.uk

www.littlebrown.co.uk

For my mother and father

I

I

Dear Reader,

There may exist a graceful and elegant way to begin one's gynecologic and colorectal memoir, but it never does spring to mind.

Let us start then with a story. We can travel back to where it all began, and for a moment leave the particulars behind. That sounds much nicer—lovely even—considering it all began so many years ago with a cool, luxuriant swim in Walden Pond.

~

I remember it well. The heat was heavy, I was a summer student at Harvard with no air-conditioning, and Walden beckoned for the reasons it always will. Though I suppose the busloads of tourists beached on the imported sand should have sounded some instinctive alarm when I arrived, they didn't. I walked right on past and made my way to the side of the pond where the water was still and the snorkelers out of sight.

I remember walking into the water. I remember floating on my back. I remember the coolness and the peace and the poetry of the place, and I remember feeling like I couldn't ask for anything more.

The next day in the emergency room, I had quite forgotten all of that.

A urinary tract infection, known as a UTI, is a very painful but easily treatable infection of the urethra. Most people describe it as "peeing broken glass," and I would have to agree with most people.

But my ER doctors patted me on the back as they ordered up the standard antibiotics and I bounded off to the pharmacy, clutching my prescription, counting the minutes in the twenty-four hours they told me it would take to go away.

Fifty-six hours later, I was back in the emergency room. It had not gone away.

In fact, it did not go away for six months. "How strange," the college physician said as he took my history. I had never been sexually active, which made things particularly challenging, both diagnostically and emotionally. I was a senior in college, and it was my time. I even had the right person picked out.

But the UTI stayed. We joked and called it my PUTI, or permanent UTI, and I laughed along with the rest. But in private, in the bathroom, I was profoundly unamused.

~

This prologue is typical of women like me. A simple and innocuous medical event—often with a gyno or gastro tilt—that should have resolved simply, but didn't. She thinks it is just another one of life's ups and downs, when in fact Up is about to become a distant memory.

There is a secret society of sorts that no one—not even the members—has heard of. We don't look alike, we don't dress alike, and we're from all over. There is no secret handshake, no meeting place, no cipher.

We are the women with mysterious illnesses, and we are everywhere.

~

When I went home for Christmas just outside of Washington, D.C., my parents—who are both top-notch physicians—made an appointment for me to see Washington's preeminent, top-notch urologist.

Dr. Damaskus said I seemed like a nice, normal young woman who would probably like to get back to the business of being able to pee and have sex freely, and he saw no reason why he couldn't make that happen. He determined I no longer had an active infection— and then proposed a procedure, to be done right there, that day, in the office. As he described it, he would insert a small instrument into the urethra, rip it, and this would solve the problem.

I frowned.

But Dr. Damaskus assured me it was the only option, should I want a normal life again—the gentle ripping, he explained, was more of a light stretching of the tissue, and it would interrupt the muscle spasm and break the cycle of pain. He handed me a paper gown.

I'm almost nostalgic for my naïveté. I took the gown, steeled my nerves, saddled up, and put my feet in the stirrups.

The procedure began benignly enough with a small swabbing of topical lidocaine, but in the next step a device not unlike a very small car jack was inserted in the urethra and then ratcheted out several notches until the urethra, as promised, tore. It was a blinding pain that no amount of lidocaine would dull. He peeked over the paper blanket and asked if I thought he had gone enough notches. I was crying too hard to do anything but nod. He went one more notch.

Dear, patient reader, I have not forgotten about you, or our purpose here—or the cautionary voice in the back of my head whispering something about too much information. But I think this history is important. So before we move out of this reverie, let me come quickly to the end of the beginning of our story.

That night, after Dr. Damaskus sent me hobbling back on my way, intuition's warning bell finally took up its low, steady thrum. I sat silently through dinner, and put myself to sleep early. Something was not right—something flulike, but menacing, was starting to bristle. Everything hurt, not just my urethra. My ears hurt. My teeth hurt. I fell asleep, my hands clenching and unclenching of their own accord.

When I woke, I was on the floor, quaking with rigors, drenched in sweat, and making a very bad noise. My mother was calling the hospital and dragging me toward the car. It appeared I had become septic, an infection of the bloodstream that would have ended badly if my mother weren't such a top-notch physician. We were at the hospital in minutes.

I was not witness to the miraculous save, but I heard all about it when I woke up. Top-shelf, nuclear-grade antibiotics pumped into me by the gallon, and it seemed like every doctor at Sibley Memorial Hospital came to sit by my side, making sure the doctors' daughter pulled through. I was extremely well taken care of. I was going to live. It would all be all right.

By the next day, everyone had gone back to their private practices, wishing me well, which I very much appreciated. The only problem was (and I hated to be a stickler)—I wasn't all right. I was still aching all over, badly, even though the infection was gone. I had a fever every afternoon, and intense pain all down my legs. The broken-glass pain was starting to radiate out to the surrounding muscles in the vagina, rectum, and bladder. My bowels seized up and stopped working. I itched.

"Strange," my doctors murmured, making notes. "How very strange."

They ran dozens of tests, but everything came back negative. At a loss (and at my insistence), they sent me back to school with painkillers and portable IV antibiotics. They said it would slowly all start to get better, and I believed it. When had my body ever done anything but get all better? I was ready to get back to the business of peeing and expressing my sexuality freely. I would carry my little IV from class to class if that's what it took.

But my body did not get better.

Class after feverish class, night after achy night, and morning after urethrally excruciating morning, I could not deny: it was getting much worse.

And in the most mysterious ways.

I was on so many medications and getting so sick so fast, it was like a rabbit hole had opened up beneath me—that I was falling slowly past the clocks and the candlesticks, and that my parents and doctors were peering over the edge, quietly watching me float down and away.

~

The entire point of *The Lady's Handbook for Her Mysterious Illness* is this:

It would have been helpful to know what a well-trafficked rabbit hole that was.

~

The unfortunate but innocuous series of medical events.

The gallons of antibiotics and fistfuls of painkillers.

The severe digestive issues, gynecologic issues, joint pain, itching, and fatigue.

The referrals, the specialists, the puzzlement.

The growing doctor-patient antipathy.

The dramatic health avalanche.

The clocks. The candlesticks.

The despair.

I thought I was the strangest medical case on the East Coast.

I was wrong.

~

Seventeen years later, I have become a well-known woman with a mysterious illness.

In the early years of this distinction, other women with mysterious illnesses would frequently introduce themselves to me, often at the most unexpected moments—at weddings, in elevators, or leaning across a bank of guests at a crowded Thanksgiving table—all wanting to discuss their own mysterious maladies. I just had to speak the words *candida* or *subclinical hypothyroid*—or the most potent of all, *gluten*—and three heads would rubberband in my direction. They either knew a woman with a mysterious illness, were married to a woman with a mysterious illness, or were themselves a woman with a mysterious illness. While other people grilled kebabs, we would speak discreetly and in low tones about constipation. When the daiquiri pitcher appeared from the kitchen, we would duck our heads to discuss whether or not daiquiris were gluten-free. At elegant cocktail parties, women were constantly pulling me into corners to talk about their vaginas.

You most likely know one of us already—a coworker, an aunt, a sister—some beleaguered old girl endlessly dealing with her health issues. She'll be reluctant to talk about the particulars but noticeably lacking in a solid diagnosis. Most people privately agree she actually suffers from an acute case of hypochondria.

This woman may not know it yet, but she is in the club.

~

WOMI.
wo.mi | whoa-mee | noun
A woman with a mysterious illness.

~

I had to make this word up myself. I would have preferred a committee, or a wealthy patron—whoever is in the business of naming—to do it for me, but no one volunteered. I'd also have preferred something more dignified than WOMI—something with gravity, preferably in the Latin. Something that provoked the right response, which in my case is, "Holy fucking shit." But because there is no name for what's wrong with me, people don't say holy fucking shit. They ask if I have tried green juice or positive thoughts.

Having a word helps.

Either way, I am sure you know a WOMI already. A spouse, a little sister, a cousin.

The signs are unmistakable. She is exhausted, gluten-free, and likely in possession of at least one autoimmune disease. She is allergic to ____ (everything), aching from tip to toe, digestively impaired, and on uneasy terms with her reproductive system. She is addled, embarrassed, ashamed, and inflamed.

She is one of us.

~

The following scene is unfolding in an office in your town every day, perhaps right now at this very moment:

Jane Doe crosses her ankles in the waiting room, absently turning the pages of *People* magazine. She looks around often—now at the oversize clock, now at the receptionist, now at the generic watercolors on the walls.

"Ms. Doe," a flat voice calls out. "Dr. Bowels will see you now. Second door on the left."

Jane takes a seat in the doctor's office, regarding the diplomas on the wall. On the desk stands a life-size replica of the human intestinal tract. When Dr. Bowels bustles in, he introduces himself as he looks over her chart for what is clearly the first time.

"Now, Ms. Doe," he says cheerfully. "What can I do for you?"

The interaction begins very seriously, a furious scribbling of notes, a furrowing of the brow, a lot of nodding. The usual diseases are ruled out and Jane confirms she has been tested, twice, for everything under the sun. Her primary symptoms are severe constipation, distention, and pain in the lower left quadrant of her abdomen. As the doctor pages through her thick medical file, Jane takes the opportunity to share some of the stranger nonbowel symptoms she has experienced—aching in the bones, fatigue, itching, unexplained gynecologic symptoms, memory problems, lower back pain— but the words are scarcely out of her mouth before she wishes she had kept her addenda to herself. She can see the red flags rising behind his eyes, and the note taking slowly tapers off. Before she knows it, where once Sherlock Holmes scribbled furiously, hot on the trail, bent on solving her mystery—he now leans back in his swivel chair, tip of his pen in the corner of his mouth, checking his watch. His look is saturated with understanding, for he has solved the case.

What we have here is not a rare, tropical disease, Watson. What we have here is an unhappy woman, badly in need of an antidepressant.

~

Six years went by before I was aware of the proverbial Jane Doe.

And again, I come from a family of excellent doctors. My mother, my father, my stepfather—even my grandmother was a famous endocrinologist. I am the absolute last person who should have walked off a medical cliff without so much as a Wile E. Coyote deadpan to the camera.

But this is how it always begins. The appointment with Dr. Bowels will likely be followed by a similar experience with Dr. Vulva, only to be repeated with Dr. Rheuma, who sends her on to Dr. Uro, and then Dr. Neuro, followed by Dr. Thyro, then possibly Dr. Chiro, and finally cycling back to Dr. Bowels. Since no lightbulbs have gone off over anyone's head, off she goes to Dr. Freud.

This long and expensive chain of events is not only common for this type of patient—it is the norm.

~

Now, it is well known that modern medicine all but requires doctors to think in algorithms.

That is, they think of the patient as a set of mathematical variables: $X + Y = Z$.

They look for the common signs and symptoms (X), corroborate it with evidence from the laboratory (Y), and, based on the symptoms and the evidence $(X + Y)$, conclude that the patient has a disease (Z). Straightforward, effective, efficient—it is the baseline of medical training.

This modern method doesn't waste valuable time or money with hand-holding, and it certainly does not encourage the patient to think of herself as a unique and special snowflake. No time for the fuzzy-wuzzies. The problem here is that Fuzzy-Wuzzy has come to include anything time-consuming at all, such as taking a full patient history. Fifteen minutes—which is now the average amount of time a doctor spends with her patient—aren't enough minutes to take a history of someone in the full bloom of health, let alone a very sick person, or a real survey of diet, exercise, sleep, and self-care regimens. It is considered an indulgence to assess the patient's personal and emotional landscape—especially with extras like empathy and a sense of connection or concern. A quick diagnosis and prescription is more expedient, and though this mechanical approach is not as artful as it could be—it gets the job done of seeing twenty or even thirty patients in a day, which many doctors have to do if they want to make a living and participate with insurance companies. Algorithmic thinking has become necessary just to keep the job.

Now, me personally, I'd prefer a large-hearted genius to take care of me—an empath and a mystic—a poet, a painter, a juggler, and a wonderful joke teller. I'd pay extra to hire out the mathematicians and statisticians to look at my lab numbers. But that's just me, and I won't impose my personal proclivities. It's not really the root of the problem anyway.

The real root problem here, regarding the women with mysterious illnesses, is this:

The algorithm is wrong.

There is a special suite of real and debilitating symptoms—you will hear me incant them over and over again to impress the point— that have mistakenly come to be seen as the telltale signs of a woman who can't cope with the pressures of real life.

Extreme fatigue.
Aching in the muscles and joints.
Chronic pain.
Multiple allergies.
Irritable bowels.
Frequent infections.
Endocrine problems.
Brain fog.

Just mentioning these symptoms can induce a total eclipse in the physician's mind of the original complaint. Before she knows it, Jane is being rotated out of the office (not without a stop at the billing counter), into the elevator, down to the lobby, and out onto the street—blinking in the morning light with nothing but a referral to a gynecologist and a script for Paxil.

When I find myself describing the above scenario to a gathering of women, it surprises even me to see an entire room of vigorously nodding heads.

~

For a concrete example, let's look at one of the classic mysterious illnesses, fibromyalgia. Also called fibromyalgia syndrome, or FMS, fibromyalgia is a syndrome whose chief symptoms include severe aching and pain in the joints and muscles, accompanied by pronounced fatigue and difficulty sleeping. No one definitively knows what causes fibromyalgia—it has been classified, then unclassified, and then classified again (and then unclassified) as an autoimmune disease—and there is great debate as to the actual, underlying pathology. But based on the symptoms alone, the best research estimates that at least one in fifty Americans has it, which is at least seven million people. And with small numbers at the NIH and the Mayo Clinic generating papers and studies routinely since the 1990s, fibromyalgia should be considered a real disease beyond any shadow of a doubt. I myself was extremely relieved to find out that there might be a name for the intense pain in my own joints and muscles—a set of symptoms that had always bewildered my doctors. It was also quite a comfort to finally discover a community of seven million people describing aspects of my exact same physical experience that had never been explained before.

Imagine then my surprise when all of my top-ranked doctors, one by one, with great professional sobriety, sat me down and cautioned me to stop telling people I had fibromyalgia.

Fibromyalgia, they explained, is just code for Crazy.

~

For years, I thought Jane Doe's situation was unique to me. My own repeated disappointment at doctor after doctor, and all because my disease was either too weird, or too unimportant. It wasn't exactly chronic fatigue syndrome (a bit too gastric, and much too pelvic), but it didn't appear to be any of the known gastroenterological or gynecologic diseases either. It was also monumentally more painful than anyone could explain. The diagnosis of fibromyalgia had been swept under the rug to preserve my credibility, and repeated colonoscopies and biopsies revealed it wasn't a known inflammatory bowel disease like ulcerative colitis or Crohn's.

Despite a truckload of symptoms, it appeared I had nothing at all.

And so maybe, since so many doctors seemed to quietly think so, it was hard not to start to think it was a simple matter of depression after all. How could they *all* be wrong? Never mind that antidepressants made me more depressed when I tried them. Never mind having built an all-around wholesome life despite my debilitating illness. And never mind my winning disposition and famously positive thoughts. If so many doctors were independently questioning my psychological composure, perhaps there was something to it.

~

I was just starting to believe this when I met my first WOMI. Her name was Charlotte.

We were brought together by our respective boyfriends at the time, and we sat for an afternoon at her small kitchen table. Piece by piece she unfolded before me the patchwork story of her own mysterious illness. As I listened I went absolutely pale, looking at her as I would a secret twin, separated from me at birth, reunited at last. Her story was so familiar—eerily familiar. I had never heard myself described to myself before. The mortal exhaustion. The urinary nightmare. The distended belly. The disaster in the pelvis. The distinct feeling of being eighty years old, despite being officially twenty-five. I could not believe I had met someone so identically strange.

But then it wasn't very long afterward that I met Naomi, a friend of my brother's, who regaled me with the story of her own mysterious illness over the telephone. A Silicon Valley mogul, Naomi had become sick with a virus when she was thirty-two, immediately became bedridden, hidden away from society for years, unable to digest anything, allergic to most of her pantry, aching all over, and prescribed enough Valium to sedate a rhinoceros.

And as she spoke, I thought:
Oh my God. Secret *triplets*.

What incredible fortune that I would meet the only two others in the whole wide world forsaken with the same wretched curse.

But then of course I would soon come to meet Sydney and then Alexandra and Skye and Christina—followed by Gwen and then Greta and then Mara and then Jones—who all, to my ever-lessening surprise, recounted almost the exact same story as my own. Varying types of related-sounding illnesses, and varying levels of severity—but undeniably variations on a very distinct theme—over and over again, almost the exact same story of the misdiagnoses, the medications, the disbelief, the rabbit hole, the Caterpillar, the Hatter, and the Hare.

And every single one of them thought they were the only one.

After about twenty of these identical conversations, the pen on my desk stirred to life and this book began to write itself.

2

At the very beginning of my research, observing WOMIs in the wild with a pair of binoculars and field notes—I was overwhelmed. No two WOMIs were alike. The number of illnesses that qualified as Mysterious was staggering. Lyme, post-treatment Lyme disease syndrome, candida, Epstein-Barr, Ehlers-Danlos, polycystic ovary syndrome, subclinical hypothyroid, dysautonomia, irritable bowel syndrome, fibromyalgia, chronic fatigue syndrome, nonceliac gluten sensitivity, heavy metal toxicity, environmental illness, sick building syndrome—I had started out with the intention of exploring intestinal health as it relates to chronic fatigue and women's health, but as soon as I turned on my headlamp, like giant moths to a tiny flame, WOMIs of all kinds came hurtling out of the jungle.

And to my surprise—far outnumbering the wholly mysterious—there was another very particular subgroup of sick women who kept thunking down out of the trees in front, behind, and next to my workstation as I tried to taxonomize the mysterious.

First there was my close friend Sydney, who told me that in addition to a series of undiagnosed intestinal complaints, she also had Hashimoto's disease. Then there was Jones, another friend saddled for a decade with unexplained symptoms, who told me she also had ulcerative colitis. Both said the same thing: the Hashimoto's and the UC were crosses to bear, but even on their medications, they were limping along in their lives with an overflow of other debilitating symptoms their doctors said were unrelated or unimportant.

I could of course empathize, but I was confused. And the sheer number of women like them, thunking down around me, made me nervous. What did Sydney's Hashimoto's disease (a disease of the thyroid) (*thunk*) have to do with Jones's ulcerative colitis (a disease of the bowel) (*thunk*)? And why were they both accompanied in rapid succession by women with lupus, multiple sclerosis, and Crohn's disease (*thunk, thunk, thunk*) with questions about fatigue and brain fog and muscle pains and back pain and unusual periods? *These aren't mysterious illnesses*—I thought indignantly—*these illnesses have respectable names!* Lupus, MS, Hashimoto's, UC, Crohn's—those are all known diseases with proper names and well-sourced Wikipedia pages. (To someone without a diagnosis, things like names and reputable Internet resources are like the holy grail.) Furthermore, my friends' illnesses affected completely unrelated parts of their bodies—kidneys, myelin sheaths, thyroid, bowel. It was distracting, and I wished they would leave me alone so I could focus on the task at hand, which was already confusing enough.

But there was no ignoring them. These girls were as WOMI as they come, and they wanted to be heard. They all reported the doctor merry-go-round, the many alternative treatments tried and failed, and the inability to find a physician to take their dis-ease seriously. Like the rest of us, they suffered the medications that suppressed one symptom and created several more—not to mention the terrible invisibleness, and the experience of hearing *But You Look Just Fine!* so often they could just cry.

And then there was the most important group of details: that telltale set of symptoms that snaked like a glittering black thread through their stories—the myalgias, the fatigue, the allergies, and the bowel problems.

We were freakishly similar.
Mysterious stepsisters.
The clues were everywhere.

But no matter what I did, I could not connect the dots. I could see there was an elephant in the living room—but what was *wrong*

with the elephant, I had no idea. I paced. I pondered. I made tea.
I studied the leaves. I studied the night sky. I couldn't make sense
of it.

And then suddenly, I could.
Standing there, head back, taking in the whole cosmos—a huge,
meandering constellation came sharply into focus.

Hashimoto's, ulcerative colitis, multiple sclerosis, lupus, Crohn's,
and sometimes fibromyalgia:

All autoimmune diseases.

~

In retrospect, it's hard to believe there was ever a time I didn't
know this. We all know a cancer when we hear one. Why should this
be different?

But it most certainly was different. I had heard all of those disease names growing up—and then more and more as I began my
investigations—but I had no idea they were the same essential type
of illness. I looked into it and learned that I was not alone in my
ignorance. According to the American Autoimmune Related Diseases Association, nine out of ten people can't name an autoimmune
disease off the top of their head. Nine out of ten seemed like an awful
lot, and while this did feel like an unusual fact, I shelved it along with
all the other unusual facts and data that did not compute. (A very
crowded shelf, bowed and sagging.)

But as I continued along, researching and observing the patterns
and behaviors of my subjects—I was astounded to find in my notes
that a *lot* of the illnesses other WOMIs had come to me with were
in fact autoimmune diseases, and I had simply not known it when I
had conducted the interviews. Sjögren's. Raynaud's. Guillain-Barré.
Rheumatoid arthritis. Celiac disease. Myasthenia gravis. Type 1 diabetes.

Autoimmune, every last one.

This seemed extremely important.

Those women had sought me out—not the other way around. They self-identified as Mysterious. They knew part of their diagnosis, but they also knew there was more to it and that something was wrong that was not being explained or treated by their physicians.

Each came in private, confessional, not sure if they qualified for the book.

They suspected their Mysteriousness but couldn't be sure.

This appeared to be another devastating function of the invisibility cloak—WOMIs wandering side by side, lost even to each other.

And so in a separate tangent from my own research, I began to read about autoimmunity—and I immediately learned that there is a *huge* autoimmune epidemic on the rise. Incidences of autoimmunity have, at a very low estimate, tripled in the last thirty years.

I was truly surprised, and for a moment in time my little world seemed to make sense. I was sure I was about to crack the code.

Mysterious illnesses, somehow = autoimmunity.
Autoimmunity, somehow = mysterious illnesses.

This was a wonderful, fireworks-filled moment.

It was also very brief.

My sagging shelf of things that didn't compute was beginning to make a low whine, and when I applied my autoimmunity epiphany to see if it accounted for everything, it did not. The autoimmune piece was a clue—a big one—but as I came back to earth and returned to the full range of my research, the more I started to realize that autoimmunity didn't actually explain things very well at all.

First of all, the cause of autoimmunity is officially unknown, and I was looking to know.

Second, there is no cure—just medications to suppress symptoms and inflammation, often causing many more symptoms, which indicated to me that it is fundamentally not well understood, and I was looking to understand.

But most importantly, this magic lasso of comprehension hadn't remotely roped all the cattle, moths, elephants, or mock turtles.

For example: *I* didn't have an autoimmune disease.

For another example, chronic fatigue syndrome isn't an autoimmune disease (though the severe presentation is often considered much worse than most autoimmune diseases).

Fibromyalgia is not currently considered an autoimmune disease.

Polycystic ovary syndrome (PCOS) is an endocrine disorder.

Candida is a fungus.

Epstein-Barr is a virus.

Lyme is caused by a spirochete.

Mold illness is caused by mold.

Drat.

The only thing these very (very) different illnesses had in common was a very (very) similar story, symptom overlap, and a slew of WOMIs who had both mysterious problems as well as autoimmune diseases. It wasn't much, but it was something. I would need to continue my investigations.

~

The next clue I already knew instinctively—I have named my book after this clue—but I was vindicated when I finally looked it up. The one thing that is obvious to everyone—to me, to doctors, to skeptics—is that this massive elephant in the living room has one very clear defining trait.

This elephant is a she.

You do not need an NIH statistic to prove this, you can just look around. It's not really Uncle Bernie's problem, it's Aunt Soozy's. You know it, Soozy knows it, and so does poor Uncle Bernie.

But the NIH is on our side here, as well. Did you know:

Eighty-five percent of fibromyalgia patients are women.
Eighty-five percent of multiple sclerosis patients are women.
Ninety percent of Hashimoto's patients are women.
Eighty percent of chronic fatigue syndrome patients are women.
Seventy-five percent of Lyme patients are women.
Ninety percent of lupus patients, women.

With a few exceptions such as Crohn's disease, which affects men just slightly more, this ratio is true almost across the board. *Seventy-five percent of all autoimmune patients are female.* And for the true mystery illnesses, the disparity is even greater—often 8:1, 9:1. This should give anyone pause—not simply because there are so many diseases affecting women these days, not simply because that discrepancy is very large, but for a more serious reason:

No one seems to notice.

I am consistently surprised to find that the numbers (when I look for them) don't just confirm my suspicions—they dwarf my suspicions. The numbers, when I look for them, are sitting there, hulking, huge, unmissable, staring at me, wondering where I've been. Wondering where everyone has been.

I hope the ax doesn't grind too hard against the stone to say it, but this being far and away a Lady's problem goes a long way toward explaining why it hasn't been taken very seriously at all.

~

Then again, let's back up a few steps. Let's just say that we're not particularly moved by the gendered aspect of the problem, and that we really have so many other important issues in this world to focus on—that is, let's say we *are* going to continue to sweep these illnesses under the rug. You can't help everyone, you know.

Well, at a rate of increase since 1980 clocking in between 200 and 300 percent:

Oh darlings.

We are going to need a significantly bigger rug.

~

But let us also be crystal clear: from the beginning, I *did* want the gender clue to be the Point.

Once I had come to understand that particular piece of the puzzle, all I wanted to do was lean back—grim in all my knowingness—sighing loudly that We Just Live in a Man's World, Girls, and them's the breaks. No one cares about these diseases because they involve women and hormones and poo and lady parts—and that's more than enough to obscure the whole thing from the national conversation.

But the truth was, an exposé about the cultural and medical bias against women's bodies would not exactly be breaking news. (See: Freud, see: hysteria.) There was more than enough for a book on that subject alone. (See Barbara Ehrenreich, see: *For Her Own Good.*) And though it would certainly have made for a simpler and more satisfying thesis, it just wasn't the whole story.

But in that case, I had to keep asking myself: what *was* going on?

Why was this widespread phenomenon being treated so casually, if we were agreed not to blame the whole thing on doctors being egomaniacal, chauvinist pigs?

This was a serious question that over the course of my research would reveal a seriously complicated answer.

And so one of the first things I ever did was to come up with a clarifying Top 10 list regarding the problems contributing to the mysterious marginalization of the mystery illnesses. This list was not exactly a clue in figuring things out—but rather a series of clues making it clearer and clearer that there really was a veil tightly drawn before anyone who was trying to figure things out.

Over a decade later, the list is still as useful as ever.

Problem 1: Invisibility

Each of the chief mysterious illnesses is largely invisible, at least according to our current standards of seeing. A typical disease presents something a doctor can observe, either under the microscope or in an examination. But not these diseases. There are no tumors, no elevated blood count, no pallor. I noticed I had to catch myself many times in my interviews—a woman would open her door, and look so absolutely normal that I couldn't help but think I'd finally found the lazybones who was just exaggerating to escape from the pressures of real life. I had to remind myself that this was exactly what people thought (and still think) about me.

But if those women just had some piece of data to hold on to, some scan to hold against the backlight, to show the world the contours of her problem—that would make a huge difference. However for such symptoms as chronic pain, fatigue, and irritable bowels, there are no scans. And this brings us to a critical point that cannot be underscored enough: the available standardized tests for the mysterious illnesses are very crude. They were in 2006, when I started looking into the matter, and they still are in 2020. Sophisticated tests are produced by sophisticated research. Which brings us right to Problem 2.

Problem 2: No Research, No Funding

This is a chicken-and-egg issue. You can't get funding to research a disease that is not considered serious or real, but a disease is not likely to be considered serious or real if there is no good research or clinical trials associated with it.

Chronic fatigue syndrome is the most glaring example, the funding for which has been historically minuscule and mismanaged. Currently there are $14 million allocated for research for CFS from the government, compared to $6.3 billion for cancer research. That is, 0.2 percent. Fibromyalgia receives the same—fourteen million, a number that comes in at the very bottom ranks of what the NIH chooses to invest in every year. Even the funding allotted for all the auto-immune diseases, which outnumber the incidences of cancer, HIV/AIDS, and heart disease combined, is just $806 million, or an eighth of the cancer fund.

Interestingly, Lyme disease actually serves as a good reminder of how important research is. Lyme disease spent about thirty years as one of the chief mysterious illnesses—and the way they partially demystified it most was when they developed a better blood titer. For decades prior, most Lyme patients were often considered as hypo-chondriac as the rest of us ladies. Nowadays, Lyme is one of the first tests they run if you come in complaining of the usual mysterious problems. This could have been a lesson—that when a disease doesn't show up in the lab tests, but corresponds identically to the anecdotal evidence of thousands of other case histories, that should speak to the inadequacy of the tests, not the inadequacy of the patients.

Alas.

Now the next batch of problems we'll have to give rapid-fire, because I have an eye on the clock, and it is just about time to get back to the story.

Problem 3: Vague Symptoms

Achy? Yeah, I got aches and pains too, lady.

Problem 4: Myriad, Overlapping Symptoms

For example, mold illness, Lyme disease, and the Epstein-Barr virus—three distinct, separate problems—can have almost identical achy, fatiguey, irritable bowely symptoms, yet no two cases are ever exactly the same. Any Lyme specialist will tell you that Lyme mani-fests in a range of expressions from individual to individual—more so than most illnesses. The same is true for Epstein-Barr, mold ill-ness, and indeed, all the mysterious illnesses. There are simply so many symptoms associated with each illness, you never know which ten of the one hundred the patient is going to present with. Thus it is extremely difficult to figure out just which permutation of the problem the patient actually has, and misdiagnoses are rampant. Furthermore, the sheer number of symptoms that tend to accompany these problems—each manageable on its own, but terrible in the aggregate—is totally overwhelming for a doctor. Night sweats, acne, abdominal distention, dry eyes, lower back pain, left ovarian pain, painful periods, exhaustion, low blood pressure, dizziness, insomnia, sensitivity to dairy, sensitivity to gluten, sensitivity to nightshades, stiffness, constipation, diarrhea, constipation *and* diarrhea—

If I were a doctor, I might be running in the other direction, too.

Problem 5: Shame

If a woman's disease happens to veer in any way toward the vaginal, the urologic, or the colorectal, then she is seriously out of luck—too unpalatable for any awareness campaign, too unsexy to start a blog, too vago-uro-colo to merit a ribbon or a million-mom march. Yet these female-centric symptoms are very common with the mysterious illnesses. That means there are millions of miserable women who are not getting the care they need because they are essentially afraid to be the gynecologically squeaky wheel.

Problem 6: Bad Treatment Options

Let's say you do luck out and get a doctor on your side who wants to help. Well, the next problem is that there are almost no tried-and-true allopathic protocols that actually help. Thus, not only does the doctor have a chronically complaining patient with invisible symptoms—when he tries to take her seriously and test out some treatments, she doesn't get better. I can see where this would frustrate a doctor and put him back to square one of nonbelieving. But I can also see that sophisticated protocols are the product of sophisticated research and implementation. Sound familiar?

Problem 7: Bias

We said we would not blame chauvinist pigs—and this is true, we can't *only* blame chauvinist pigs. But to leave them out of the equation entirely would be a serious oversight. You can be sure that if 85 percent of fibromyalgia patients were men, rendering them unable to work from extreme fatigue, bone-deep pain, and mind fog—there would be no problem getting the funding and research to look into this scourge upon the modern male workforce.

And so Problem 7 brings us right to Problem 8.

Problem 8: Fear and Loathing of the Female Patient

My own father has been known to ask a certain type of chronically complaining woman if her left elbow hurts when she urinates—a completely bullshit question—and will be amused when the answer is yes. In part, this is because my father is a jokingly self-described egomaniacal chauvinist. (Note: my father is also a very caring physician, if prone to pranks and helping people take themselves less seriously.) But in part, and I hate to say it:

Some women can be very—how shall we say—*tenacious* about their health. And this tenacity is almost regardless of how healthy they are.

Believe you me.

But on the other hand, let's be fair:

Isn't it vital that someone in the family be vigilant about the family's health? While women are frequently criticized for dragging their husbands to the doctor, the truth is that women frequently save their husbands' lives. And their own lives. Not to mention that women are also much more active in making sure their children receive regular medical care and checkups, which is a good thing.

But unfortunately, this positive interpretation is not the party line. The party line is that women are irrepressibly worried about their bodies for no reason at all, and seek medical attention more often than men purely because they are the nervousest of Nellies.

Problem 9: Our Broken Health Care System

This merits an entire shelf of books unto itself (and there are of course already hundreds), but the fact remains: the American health care system is not functioning well. As noted, if you have a complex disease that is difficult to diagnose, then a fifteen-minute HMO doctor's visit and quick-fix prescription for pain medication is clearly inadequate. If you're healthy as a horse, a fifteen-minute visit is probably inadequate.

Furthermore, most medical schools do not offer almost any training in nutrition, and as we'll get into later, proper nutrition is the foundational and easiest way to prevent and sometimes reverse many chronic illnesses. Just that statement alone, *"proper nutrition is the foundational and easiest way to prevent and sometimes reverse many chronic illnesses,"* is anathema to most medical students.

But in the end, the roots of all these problems—not enough time to listen, no emphasis on healthy behaviors, and no robust systems to help patients with behavioral change—come back to the same problem.

They are not wildly profitable.

Virtually every problem in the health care system can be understood by following the money.

If something is not a cash cow, it isn't just ignored—it will often be actively campaigned and lobbied against as dangerous, indulgent, or pseudoscience. It is a sad state of affairs, but in no way a secret state of affairs, and it can't be emphasized enough.

Anyway, I promise we're coming to the end. Did I mention it's complicated?

And we have yet to talk about the most intriguing problem of all:

Problem 10: These Epidemics Are New

Fibromyalgia, chronic fatigue syndrome, multiple sclerosis, Hashimoto's disease, Lyme disease, lupus, polycystic ovary syndrome—in 1960, these were all rare. But in the last fifty years the new cases of these diseases have been raining down from the sky like hail, frogs, and locusts.

Fifty million women in this country suffer from these illnesses, at a very low estimate.

That's one in four women.

And that, girls, is a lot.

~

So this is how it began.

After several years of fieldwork in this area, I casually remarked to my friend Elena that I had begun work on a book that would be called *The Lady's Handbook for Her Mysterious Illness*. I joked that it would be a modern everywoman's tale, an Odyssean adventure—complete with mysteriously sick sirens, stethoscope-wearing cyclopses, and an epic intestinal battle. And this friend of mine had (of course) dealt with a horrible mysterious illness of her own, so she was enthusiastic. Encouraged, I went back to the business of sketching out my pet project, wrestling over important questions, like which was the best chapter title, *Yeast of Burden* or *The Red Vag of Courage*.

But then a curious thing happened—something that would happen over and over again during the next decade. By the end of that week, I received e-mails from six women I had never met. They were friends of Elena's, and they wanted to share their stories for the project. They all had mysterious maladies—from post-treatment Lyme disease syndrome to candida to chronic fatigue—and we e-mailed back and forth. And in a few weeks, as they put the word out, women started popping up everywhere, describing to me in the minutest detail the function and dysfunction of their intestinal tracts. We would compare cupboards full of supplements, occult healing modalities, and caches of our rogue research. But what they mainly wanted was for someone to listen to them, and that I could do. I listened to over two hundred women of all sorts—younger, older, richer, and poorer. I listened to stories of how their own bodies had slowly gone to pieces, or how their daughter's body was unraveling right in front of them, or how their best friend was vaguely (and often not so vaguely) deteriorating.

On my listening tour, I began to have the sense that my pet project with the joke chapter titles and the strong stances on microbiota and the patriarchy was actually the thing these women had been looking for all those lonely afternoons spent wandering Barnes & Noble, coming up empty among the self-help books, the fad diet cookbooks, and the gentle pastel books about women's health.

And I confessed to myself, it was the thing I had been looking for, too.

And this is how *The Lady's Handbook for Her Mysterious Illness* came to pass—a book designed for aunts, coworkers, sisters, and girlfriends alike—a book to keep under her pillow late into one of her dismal, insomniac nights—a book to share with her support group, or family, or book club—a book bearing a very simple message:

You are not crazy.

And most important, you are not alone.

3

As it turns out, a "Walden" of some kind is very common, found in nearly every case history of a WOMI. There is almost always some kind of triggering event.

A rape.
A trauma.
A divorce.
A death.
A virus.
An accident.

The journey begins when the earth cracks wide and down she goes.

And for your narrator, it was no different.

Walden.
The PUTI.
Dr. Damaskus.
Septic shock.
The emergency room.

Goodbye, Sarah.
Goodbye, WOMIs.

And good luck.

~

Next, as a woman like me begins to descend—blue dress belled around her—she is innocent, unaware that the rules of reality are now and forever reversed. When she touches the ground, up is now down, and left is now right. Riddles abound.

Medically speaking, the woman is supposed to be getting better and better, but she is getting worse. Where this formerly ambitious young woman once stayed up late in the stacks studying religion and philosophy and literature, or stayed up late running a company, or running a family, or running for office—or all of the above—now she is glued to her bed for most of the day, immobile, drifting in and out of sleep.

When she does sleep, she wakes only to discover she is more tired.
When food goes in, it now declines to come out.
She looks normal, but she feels like the walking dead.

Whatever the expectation may be, reality is now inverted.

For example:

After the Incident with Dr. Damaskus, I returned to college under a heavy and invisible blanket of illness. I carried my portable IV antibiotics with me in a cooler, and my roommates sat with me in rocking chairs while I shot liquid antibiotics into my arm. I rolled between classes and bed and back to classes like a wet log, waking with a start, to find I had been dead asleep, face-first on my desk in a class called "The Amazing Brain."

Furthermore, where illnesses had always been upfront and honest with me before—announcing their comings and goings with trumpets and checkered flags—now illness was very coy.

Now my health was a trickster, a shapeshifter, a shroud, a mist.
Now my symptoms were vague and diffuse, tapping me on the shoulder, only to dematerialize every time I turned around.

Aches, pain, fatigue, brain fog, digestive upset, general malaise.

Now it was everywhere and nowhere at once.

~

In the face of a mysterious illness, Western protocol is to break it down and attack it piece by piece—separating the vaginal from the gastrointestinal from the rheumatalogical.

But because the mysterious illnesses affect multiple body systems, this approach doesn't work very well, and an enormous number of disjointed appointments need to be made. While other people go through their hectic daily life, a WOMI's life becomes hectic-bordering-on-mania, spent continuously propping herself up with stimulants and food, whilst wedging in appointments between the already-full units of the modern daily grind.

While no one can see it, being sick is like taking a second job in secret twenty-, thirty-, sixty-minute increments throughout the day, hidden from view.

My case was no different.

And I'll mention this one last time: virtually all of my parents are doctors. Mother, father, stepfather, plus the famous grandmother. I was the last person who should have fallen into a medical black hole.

But, down and down I went.

In between classes, and on spring break, and then long after I graduated—instead of being a young person and setting out on the voyage of life, my rectum was being probed, vagina splayed, bladder catheterized, barium enemas administered, sticky "anal paddles" applied, heart monitored, IVs hooked and unhooked, lines threaded and unthreaded.

I saw all the best doctors, in every possible field, at every possible beacon of modern medicine on the East Coast. I underwent every MRI, CAT scan, PET scan, transvaginal ultrasound, transesophageal echocardiogram, and black dye contrast study catheterization available—often three or more times. We tested for parasites and rare diseases, from babesiosis to dengue fever. I took course after course of top-shelf antibiotics, muscle relaxants, pain medications, birth-control pills and patches, and finally antianxiety medication and antidepressants—all in exchange for the steady decline in my health. In fact, all of this testing and drugging seemed to drive the disease deeper into my system.

Questions upon questions.
Answers begetting more questions.
Total professional embafflement.

The result: ever more tests, scopes, scans, probes, samples, swabs.

No stone left unswabbed.

Urologist A would cross all the major concerns off his list, and suggest seeing gastroenterologist B. Gastroenterologist B would run all available tests and rectal probings, cross all major concerns off his list, and suggest seeing gynecologist C. Gynecologist C would perform her excruciating manual examination, cross all the major concerns off her list, and suggest going back to urologist A.

Around and around and around—a caucus race with no beginning and no end.

One could say it is the patient, not the illness, that is progressively broken down.

~

So what exactly *was* wrong, with me specifically? An excellent question, one we all had a lot of trouble answering. Because as you will see—it was not just one problem, but a laundry list of problems. Thus, here I need to present to you the mess my doctors were presented with—a graphic exercise I'll ask you to bear with this one time to give the fullest possible picture of my odd, complex illness.

And I should probably note: mine is odder, and more complex, than most.

And significantly more vaginal.

~

The first order of business was straightforward enough, and this was to address the Incident.

Obviously "it" had started there, with Dr. Damaskus—and while it did eventually seem like something must have gone wrong, what that thing was, no one could guess. This was complicated by the fact that Dr. Damaskus did not indicate that there had been any wrong-doing. And so all we were left with were the facts that the procedure had been indescribably painful (which it should not have been), that I had bled quite a bit afterward (which is not normal for this procedure), and that I had become septic (which clearly indicated something gone wrong). There were also several subsequent scans—PET, CAT—and transvaginal ultrasounds that showed a small abnormality on the left side of the vagina.

However, nothing could be extrapolated definitively from this evidence.
The vagina is so nerve-rich, dense, and complex, it is notoriously difficult to image.

There wasn't enough data to say *this*, this is the problem.

And because nothing definitive could be extrapolated, and because Dr. Damaskus indicated everything had gone to plan, all this evidence was quickly deemed irrelevant, moved to the bottom of the pile, and forgotten.

Which left us with a procedure deemed totally normal.
Which left us with a patient experiencing an unusual, grossly outsized reaction.

And so, right from the beginning, we were not off to a great start.

~

The second order of business was to catalog that unusual, out-sized reaction.

A very, very long catalog.

Number one on the list was the issue of pain. At first it was just simple pain in and around the left side of the vagina, from the fiery to the stabbing, as well as burning pain on the left side of the bladder, the urethra, and the vagina. But as time went on, this would snowball into extreme pain and spasm in all of the pelvic floor muscles, including those in the whole of the vagina, the rectum, the sacrum, the groin, the hip flexor region, the urethra, the bladder, the uterus, the cervix, and the left ovary. And as even more time went on, this pain would only get worse, spreading up the spine, throughout the left side of the abdomen, and down the left leg.

Number two on the list was the issue of the bowel. At the time of the Incident and the subsequent flood of antibiotics, my bowel had simply stopped evacuating. Like, finito. No bowel signals or peristalsis at all—it just shut down, as if it had been put to sleep—and no prune, no fiber, no extra hydration, no MiraLAX, and no stool softener could make it wake up again. The only thing that worked was to take quadruple the dose of laxatives a normal person might take—and this did make the bowels empty, but at the cost of now having daily, explosive diarrhea. However, because even a single day of not pooping would create an unbearable pressure on the already red-hot nerves in my spine and bladder and vagina (pressure that mysteriously caused the left labia minora to swell to even more unspeakable proportions), I had to take the laxatives. This started to create a vicious cycle, and the bowel became ever more dependent on the laxatives—but I couldn't stop, because every time I tried, the pain was unbearable. I began to have to do enemas or take as much laxative as a colonoscopy prep—every single day—just to empty the colon and relieve the pressure on those fiery nerves.

But a mutinous colon was only the tip of the gastrointestinal iceberg. As the illness progressed, I began to develop extreme pain in the stomach upon eating anything at all. I also started to exhibit a permanently distended stomach, which wrenched and twisted in pain virtually all the time. Every time I ate anything, from pad Thai to a handful of blueberries, my eyes would start to water, my ears itched, and my nose ran—despite never having had a single food sensitivity in my life. My pyloric sphincter, much like my internal anal sphincter, stopped opening and closing properly—and this stricture made the passage of food from the stomach to the small intestine quite painful.

Then, there was the issue of the more classically Mysterious symptoms. As the snowball rolled along, my symptom cloud grew larger and larger—now including terrible itching every time I ate sugar, bloating, extreme fatigue, night sweats, brain fog, and a furry tongue. There were unexplained fevers, all the time, and I slept constantly. And the worse it got, the weirder it got. There was an intermittent, honking bronchial cough, and serious radiating pain in my upper spine, which is called radiculitis (pronounced *ridiculitis*, which I thought was actually a rather good name for the whole disease). I was also experiencing frequent yeast infections and bacterial vaginosis. And in addition to incapacitating menstrual cramps and cystic ovaries, I would often vomit and black out when my period came. I also seemed to exhibit all the signs of fibromyalgia (a deep aching and pain in the muscles and bones that came in flares) as well as a huge array of new sensitivities to detergents, moldy basements, cigarette smoke, and strong chemical fumes—something called multiple chemical sensitivity. I developed trouble standing up for long periods of time, and would become dizzy, with a racing heartbeat, and extremely tired after exerting myself the slightest amount—something called POTS, or postural orthostatic tachycardia syndrome, though I was not diagnosed with that at the time. And if all this were not enough, when I was given pain medications and muscle relaxants and birth-control pills (from Tylenol 3 to Skelaxin to Flexeril to Neurontin to tramadol to codeine to Ortho-Cyclen), I became nauseated, achy, and somnolent to the point of barely being conscious—something called "a paradoxical reaction."

Altogether, the whole strange thing seemed to have avalanched into something mimicking a weird autoimmune disease of some kind—as if things had been going so badly for so long, my body had relearned its own status quo, and the new normal was to set off all the alarms, all the time, even if the intruder was long gone.

And it's important to note that somehow, after listening to this mini Armageddon of symptoms, sometimes all my doctors ended up writing in the chart was:

"Chronic fatigue syndrome."

And I think this is perhaps because of the most complicating factor of all:

I looked (and still look) almost 100 percent normal.

Great even. I glow.

Especially later on, after I cut out wheat, dairy, sugar, and started doing yoga. Not only was I slightly radiant but, because of the pain in my central cavity, I was always, always in some kind of flowing, pretty dress. More than a few doctors implied that whatever seemed to be the problem—it suited me.

This is one of the biggest psychological tormentors of the invisibly ill: the disconnect between the way you feel and the constant refrain from family and friends that you look just fine. I am sure it partly explains how for seven of the thirteen years all this was going on, not a single diagnosis from that extensive list I just rattled off was anywhere be seen. I was just a walking thicket of complaints— with an expanding accordion file documenting what it was Not. My mostly healthy-looking exterior (not to mention sunny personality) didn't help, but the trouble was also that my doctors were intent on coming up with a name—the one and true name that would succinctly explain all the many bizarre and disparate problems my body seemed to house under one roof. And, of course, I wanted this too. Occam's razor. A label. A name.

But unfortunately, what we had on our hands was the illness that has no name.

~

Without a name, and without a medical stamp of approval, all a woman with a mysterious illness is left with is a truckful of symptoms, a world full of raised eyebrows, and just barely muted judgments. After exceeding the normal threshold of time to find a diagnosis and coming up empty, the innocence that defines the initial descent starts to dissipate and her new life slowly reveals itself to be a kind of waking nightmare. Not only is she sick, no one believes her.

The same can be seen in the case of an illness that has an unserious name—and in the land of the mysteriously ill, these names abound. Irritable bowel syndrome, sick building syndrome, mold illness, yeast, leaky gut syndrome, and of course the most dreaded of all, chronic fatigue syndrome.

Which is also, just to underscore the point, colloquially known as:
The Garbage Pail Syndrome.

Obviously, none of these conjure a sense of importance or empathy, and to everyone except the chronic fatigue syndrome sufferer, "chronic fatigue syndrome" is a phrase generally employed with an emphasis on the air quotes.

And this low opinion isn't just true for laypeople. The same view will surface with many of this patient's future doctors, who slowly look up and over their spectacles when she mentions her "chronic fatigue syndrome." Once that unwanted cat is out of the bag, all hopes for a partnership with the new doctor are often dashed. A change can be seen in real time coming over the heath care provider—and this phenomenon is true for WOMIs across the board, from those with subclinical thyroid problems to those with unexplained perimenopausal problems, fatigue problems, memory loss, pooping problems—all of it is rejected by the algorithm, which stares back at her, green cursor blinking slowly on the screen. She inserts the floppy disk of her feelings, thoughts, and experiences—all these many symptoms, and how terribly they are affecting her life, and how concerned she is to be so young and so broken down—and the computer simply continues to stare back, blinking.

Input Denied.

She stammers and tries to explain. What about these thirteen symptoms—and these activities like sex, and sitting, and reading, which she can no longer do, and the terrible way she feels upon waking, and the pain in her joints? The ovarian cysts, the pelvic pain, the scoliosis, the constipation, and the—

Input Denied.

The more she talks, the less response she gets.

And if she does turn out to have something diagnosable, like PCOS or lupus or MS, the situation does not very much improve. She is told that PCOS, lupus, and MS have no cure, only symptom management—and unfortunately, the symptom management notoriously causes almost as many symptoms as the disease itself.

But ultimately, if she doesn't have a diagnosable illness, well, you may by now suspect what is coming next.

~

In my case, the physician who finally came up with the solution that stuck was Manhattan's preeminent urologist. We'll call him Dr. Urethra.

After a brief consultation about the situation, he decided on a strange and painful procedure to look for a urethral diverticulum— that is, an abnormal outpouching next to the urethra that can contain bacteria, and could somewhat explain the Dr. Damaskus debacle. Eight electrical nodes were pasted to my already-burning inner buttocks, a huge shot of antibiotics was administered to my outer buttocks, and a catheter was inserted roughly up my unanesthetized, flaming-hot, burning urethra.

This catheterization produced tears, and those tears produced a very aggravated Dr. Urethra.

After padding down the hallway with my dangling tubes and wires in hand, I was seated on a rubber toilet seat attached to a machine that raised me four feet into the air, my paper gown open and flapping in the back. Then a small convoy of observers—the doctor, an intern, a nurse, and a technician—all huddled and watched a screen, where an image of my bladder began to fill with black contrast dye. And as we all looked on, I was supposed to say "When" when my bladder felt full. So we all watched with interest as the balloon grew bigger and bigger and bigger and bigger—until Dr. Urethra started swiveling his head between me and the screen, his eyes wide, prompting me to "Say when," "Say when!" But the signal for "When" wasn't coming, I didn't feel the need to pee—and instead the room started to go dark, and the doctor started shouting, and a wave of nausea crashed over me—and I proceeded to faint, slumping off the aerial, rubber, mechanized toilet seat, onto the intern, gracelessly losing my paper gown.

I was awakened with smelling salts, and the first person I saw was Dr. Urethra, pacing, red in the face, grumbling, and quite angry. He appeared to be upset that I had bungled the test. Seeing this, and still very much, and very painfully catheterized, I started to cry again. I couldn't help it. But this second round of tears decisively broke the camel's back, and Dr. Urethra stormed out.

After the nodes and the tubes and the gown had been removed, the nurse called my family into the office. Dr. Urethra had composed himself, and proceeded to explain in even tones that while the test was difficult to pull off, he had been able to get what he needed—and found nothing, no diverticulum, no sign of anything unusual whatsoever.

Furthermore—he said, removing his glasses and speaking now directly to my parents and not to me—from what he could gather from our experience together, he had concluded that my problem, "like many young women her age," was psychological.

I was awarded a clean bill of health and sent on my way.

~

I never saw Dr. Urethra again. For all he knows, I went into therapy and was cured. I think this is very common—doctors never see or hear again from the patients they shame, and so there is no way to feel or see how damaging, and incorrect, their behavior is.

But the big problem was not Dr. Urethra in isolation.

He is forgiven, and we more or less wish him the best.

For any WOMI, the problem we face isn't the one errant jerk of a doctor who happens to decide we need to have our head checked instead of receiving medical care. Jerky behavior isn't optimal, surely, but we're big girls. We can take it.

The real problem is how painfully common that exchange with Dr. Urethra turns out to be.

That exchange isn't a one-off mistake.

That exchange, for people like me, is protocol.

Again and again and again (but not without a stop at the billing counter), doctor after doctor reached a hand inside of me, rooted around, caused me extraordinary, blinding pain—and if this produced any emotional response whatsoever, the entire appointment was washed away by a river of my own tears. If they couldn't find a diagnosis, or a lump, or something tangible—and when I persisted in looking so confounded normal, except that I sometimes cried or looked unhappy—instead of saying, "Well, we don't know, but let's keep trying," they all began to recommend psychiatric counseling.

Again. And again. And again.

(See: *If These Vaginal Walls Could Talk*.)

I'm not antitherapy or anti-antidepressant—I have adored certain therapists, and know many people who have been helped by antidepressants. And I'm not saying I wasn't emotional or at times very sad. Of course I was—I had a hideous vaginal disease. But the notion that my sadness would drive me to misperceive or make up something so . . . elaborate (not to mention humiliating) (not to mention rectal) as a cry for help—well, this was quite a shock.

Mostly, it just didn't stand to reason. Even if no one believed me about the aching and the itching and the pelvic pain—which, I get it, you can't see on a scan or under the microscope—there was still hard evidence of something wrong. The fevers. The soccer-ball stomach. The swollen labia. The furry tongue.

It didn't matter.

In the end, I caved, and even my parents got on board. With my consent, my father was the one to write me my first prescription for Paxil.

~

I have always thought the best subtitle for this book would be: *The Lady's Handbook for Her Mysterious Illness: A Cautionary Tale.*

4

About a year into things, I grew a second self.

It was an exterior self that I would present to the world—someone who smiled and did fabulous things and did not have a fire poker in her vagina, bladder, intestines, and spinal cord. This second self is so, so very common with the Ladies. When no one can see or understand the disease, even in a basic way, things get complicated. She is afraid of being stigmatized, so she stops talking about it. She may take significant time off, change her eating habits, take naps—and sometimes this produces real, positive change. But usually she feels guilty for taking this time for her made-up disease, and comes back to the world with a zealous but not totally genuine zest for life—instantly burning out any energy she might have cultivated during her resting period.

I can't stress how typical this is. While there are indeed some women who are hypochondriacs, and some women who do complain incessantly about their problems to anyone who will listen—and alternatively, there are some women who are so bedridden, so immediately and so catastrophically that this avatar life does not apply (see: severe chronic fatigue syndrome)—in my observation these poles are the distinct minority. Most are in the silent, secret majority.

And so in the beginning, the partially healed WOMI applies for big-time jobs, works long hours, or tries to start her own business so she can work from home, attempting to keep up the facade of success, or at least the facade of positivity. It is exhausting, but in the end, she thinks to herself dourly that at least she has an impressive résumé.

Three of the first mysteriously ill women I ever encountered were superstars this way: two were *New York Times* bestselling authors and one had sold her hugely successful Internet start-up for $30 million.

All while they were sick.

I was exactly the same way.

And we are all agreed: there simply comes a point when you decide that if it is going to be so outrageously bad on the inside, and there is no cure, you will try to create something outrageously good on the outside.

So that's what I did.

In 2004, I was given a break. A pretty big one, actually. After months spent staring into the infinite abyss of the family couch pillows, unable to read or even sustain conversation—my doctor mother went rogue and prescribed me Diflucan for a basic yeast infection I had, on the one condition that I not tell my doctors. She had suspicions that a fungal infection might be driving the whole illness—and in alternative medicine, candida, or a systemic, subclinical yeast infection of the intestines, is a common but very controversial diagnosis. In traditional Western medicine, this Phantom Fungus Syndrome is widely regarded as a condition that only kooks and hypochondriacs believe in, and absolutely does not exist.

And at that point in my journey, this poor opinion of candidiasis was just fine with me. I myself did not like to think my problem was "yeast." Ew.

But I took the medication anyway—and lo, readers:

A miracle.

After months and months of severe lethargy, cemented bowels, the foggiest brain, and extreme vaginal pain—your Sarah Ramey was raised from the dead, suddenly much better, from head to toe, within about a week. The pain receded some, the fever evaporated, and my energy started to return. I could *read*.

Free at last, free at last! I didn't waste any time with the important things, and lost my virginity almost immediately.

Painful? Oh God.
But it was possible.

I.
Was.
Ecstatic.

I was a nice, normal young woman again.

And this supreme enthusiasm is just as common as common can be. An average WOMI's reentry into what she thinks will be normal life as she has always known it can be characterized with phrases like "wild abandon" and "devil may care." It is the equal and opposite reaction to months sewn into the sheets of her bed in suspended, horizontal animation.

And, importantly, she may also take up a campaign to disassociate herself from all signs of weakness. Her illness *will not* be a stain on her reputation. She is not a failure. And she will make sure of this, even if she has to lock certain things away—symptoms, feelings, needs—like a telltale heart, thumping in the basement. This behavior is regardless of the severity of whatever syndrome she is dealing with. One WOMI I know calls this the "boom/bust cycle," and it is so very understandable. Because in the beginning, a WOMI has no idea what is going on, and certainly does not see her body as a temple. That concept is just not part of our culture. Her body is a vehicle that gets her brilliant head from one location to another. She is calmly aware she might be driving a lemon, but when the thing begins to show real signs of wear, she has learned to bang the dashboard and use her force of will to keep it moving—no matter what. Her answer to a sputtering car is to floor it.

And this is exactly what I did.
Given an inch, I took a thousand miles.

~

Immediately following my partial resurrection:

I moved to Maine.
I lived by the ocean.
I waitressed.
I had a boyfriend.
I had sex.
I joined a band.
We toured the country.
I seized the day.
I seized the night.
And seeing that I was doing well, I was taken off the medication after six months, because there is legitimate concern that long-term use of prescription antifungals is dangerous to the liver.

And then I ignored/hid/locked in the basement the signs that I was ever so slowly starting to get worse again. Because who could really believe that fungus could have anything to do with my problem?

But more than that, I was terrified of getting back on the medical merry-go-round.

So instead:

I tried to be one of the guys.
Strong.
Tough.
Machine.
Coffee.
Beer.
Pizza.
I would lie curled up in the backseat of our van, outside some bar in Idaho, waiting for a gig to start, praying for poop.

When sex became excruciating again, I silently bit my lip.

When I was hospitalized for constipation, I told no one.

When my body started to ache and burn, I made myself join a gym.

I could not, would not go back to the mechanical, medical nightmare.

Thus:

I applied instead to Columbia University's MFA program for creative writing, and got in.

I moved to New York.

I started writing a biography of my endocrinologist grandmother.

I started dating a sensitive male model.

The male model brought me offerings of feathers, seashells, and gluten-free delicacies, set before me as if they were frankincense, gold, and myrrh.

All of this seemed like good medicine.

And yet:

I got much, much worse.

It felt like I had poured cement into my colon and put a hatchet in my vagina.

The fevers returned.

I became allergic to everything.

And I mean *everything*.

I lost twenty pounds in two months, and I was skinny to begin with.

I had to give myself suppositories in the ladies' room.

I sat in class, trying to focus on Vladimir Nabokov, John McPhee, and Virginia Woolf, closing my eyes to do quiet, Lamaze-style breathing just to get through sitting for two hours in a wooden chair.

No one knew.

I finally started going secretly to gastroenterologists, urologists, rheumatologists, by myself.

And I found myself universally prescribed antidepressants and antianxiety medications.

I didn't know what to do.

Every single doctor had the same diagnosis: female sadness.

I broke under the weight of my secret and told my family, three friends, and the model.

I was embarrassed and emaciated.

I was urged to drop out of school.

I agreed instead to start Paxil and Klonopin.

Then:

I had three energetic weeks, zooming around on some much-needed serotonin, pooping like a champion—until suddenly without any warning I fell into the blackest, bleakest hole of true, crushing depression and started to plan my own suicide, all day, every day.

I started having severe panic attacks—on the subway, in my room, at school.

I told my doctors, and my doctors told me to increase the Klonopin (a sedative) and find a therapist.

I went to a psychologist, who listened to my story from beginning to end, and all but kicked me out of her office, demanding I get real medical attention.

I didn't know what to do.

I stopped writing about Grandma, and started writing about my vagina.

I presented this writing to my workshop.

They liked it.

It was a cold comfort.

The model and I broke up.

I slept constantly.

I couldn't eat anything without my stomach blowing up like a balloon.

I had to walk very slowly.

I could no longer sit in a chair.

I barely graduated.

And so:

I went on the lam.

Immediately after graduation, I moved into our family's small summer cabin, alone.

The house sits at the end of Solitary Lane.
The porch overlooks Solitary Creek.
This is true.

Just before leaving, I had met a yoga teacher named Alejandro del Sol—my first encounter with yoga—who had given me a gentle practice I could do on my own. I had also met my first fellow WOMI by this point, the secret twin, who advised me to attend to my gut flora, and go on a paleo diet (no sugar, no grains).
These were two blessed, much-needed rays of Sol.
Retreating into Solitary, I did exactly as they said, every day.
And I started to get a little better.
At my twin's urging, I started taking herbal antifungals.
And I got a little bit better.
At Alejandro's urging, I planted a small garden.
At everyone's urging, I stopped taking the antidepressants.
The suicidal thoughts vanished.

And slowly, I got a little better.
And then a little better.

But I was still extremely isolated.
And I was definitely still sick, just a bit better.

I took up meditating.
I took up prayer.
I prayed for something, anything, to come in and save me from the invisible monster.

And then one day, after very slowly improving over a few months, a friend called and told me about a job opening at Barack Obama's campaign headquarters in Chicago. It was August of 2007 and they needed a blogger. They needed someone who could write fast, and move right away. It was ludicrous for someone in my situation to apply. I applied.

Two weeks later, I had an apartment in Chicago, and an average readership of 25,000 people a day.
I absolutely loved it.

I wrote about Hope and Change every day.

I had brilliant colleagues, straight off the set of *The West Wing*.

My own hope engine came back online, and my wasted heart started to beat.

We worked sixteen-hour days.

We worked seven days a week.

I was happy.

I met Barack Obama.

I edited a few lines of his speeches.

I read the "Yes We Can" speech in a Word document the night before it came out.

And:

I was unbelievably sick.

The chasm between public me and private me was immense.

I had to wake at four-thirty in the morning to give myself the first of two morning enemas, stretch my pelvic floor, make all of my own food and laxative tea, do yoga, pray and meditate—just so I could keep myself functioning enough to do the job.

I couldn't wear pants, and had to sit at a forty-five-degree angle on my thigh to keep all weight off my pelvis.

I ached like I was 128 years old, not 28 years old.

I cried every day in the campaign headquarters bathroom, crouching in the stall.

I slept in my car on breaks.

And I kept it all a secret.

I loathed keeping it a secret.

I loved these friends.

I loved my job.

My friends and my job loved me back.

It didn't matter.

By the Iowa caucuses, I was so crippled from pain and exhaustion that I could barely walk to the bathroom to cry.

I was flown home for emergency intestinal surgery and could not go back to Chicago.

My emergency laparoscopy revealed nothing except a "flaccid colon."

A flaccid colon, it turns out, is nothing to worry about.

I saw more specialists. I was tested for everything, again.

I was told everything was normal, again.

I was told I could either Botox the muscles in my vagina, which probably wouldn't do a whole lot, or I could start making preparations for dealing with my imagined condition permanently.

~

Writing this now, I want to reach through the screen and pull my younger self close.

I am so, so sorry. I didn't know.

~

I did not Botox my vagina.

A slow realization—starting at Columbia, continuing through my monkish period in Solitary, and then dramatically when I returned home from Chicago—had been dawning on me for some time: when it came to my body, no one had any idea what they were doing. This was really a new thought. It had never occurred to me that even though I had doctor parents, they might not eventually figure out how to help. Gaunt and quiet in my sickbed, I watched my father and mother pore over the medical literature, looking for some way to save their daughter. But all the solutions they could find—more medications and more surgeries—were just grasping at straws, and straws with high risk for further damage or complications, considering we did not know or understand what was causing the problem in the first place. I was not about to inject botulinum toxin into my vagina, or have my bowel resected, or have a spinal cord stimulator implanted, considering the total absence of any diagnosis, and that just taking Tylenol 3 sent me spiraling in horrific paradoxical reactions.

But they were desperate.
They had a wild look in their eye.
So did I.

And so when the call came in late May of 2008 from a friend of
the family I had never met—that beautiful millionaire whose Internet start-up was such a success—and she wanted to talk to me about
her experience with her own mysterious disease, I was all ears. She
was sitting at lunch in San Francisco with my brother, who had just
told her my story. She had picked up his phone and called me herself.

After twelve years of a completely debilitating, completely mysterious illness—one that had been made worse by Western treatment, one that had sent her into a monk's existence for years, one
that had been a major factor in driving her to become an Internet
mogul as a demonstration of strength, and one that had finally forced
her to quit working—she had found an extraordinary acupuncturist. Her acupuncturist was famous. This woman had brought many
people I'd heard of back from the almost dead. She had brought the
beautiful millionaire back from the almost dead.

"If I were you, and I know this sounds dramatic, I would pack
your bags and move to San Francisco."

Two weeks later, I was on a plane heading for California.

5

For any WOMI who has been plummeting in free fall—perhaps for years—finally unlatching the door into alternative medicine is like walking through the wardrobe. This is the beginning of the famed Health Journey—an increasingly well-known, portentous journey of our time. The rise of the health movement and alternative modalities are difficult to miss—they are everywhere, and everyone seems to be healing—and there is little doubt that the number one customer driving the zeitgeist is Jane Doe. Ideas such as food being used as medicine, herbs instead of medications, a subtle energetic system in the body, and emotions contributing in a real way to illness—these ideas start to make small tears in the fabric of a WOMI's reality, where she gets glimpses and intimations that life as she has known it—the doctors, the coldness, the scoping, the scanning, and also the pizza, the beer, the Diet Coke, the Twizzlers—might, *might,* not be all there is to know.

And after years of traditional health care that may have been unhelpful or damaging to her morale and sense of worth, the notion of quality holistic health care can feel like a kind of extraordinary homecoming. The hearth fires are lit, everyone is kind and happy to see her, and there is a real sense she is supposed to be there. They believe her! Her whole body is taken in by one practitioner—no need to see a different specialist for every organ. She is accepted as an entire, valid being.

But more than simple acceptance—she is finally getting treatment that has a steady, positive impact on her health. For the weary traveler, whose experiences may have been extremely negative, cold, and diminishing—with a steady, adverse impact on her health—this kind of care is a warm, bright shelter in the storm.

This marks a completely new stage of her experience.

Before, she was falling, falling, falling—drugged deeper and deeper and deeper—sometimes rising, but always buffeted about by chance. But now, something deep inside has woken up, and in this stage, regardless of how sick, she will begin to gather documents, scientific studies, health books, and wisdom from the worlds of traditional Chinese medicine, Ayurveda, herbalism, yoga, naturopathy, and not a few Zen Buddhists. There are many areas to explore—the meridians, the chakras, the psyche, the diets, the fascia, the bowel flora—which is overwhelming, but engrossing. She is a health detective, and she will apply everything in the laboratory of her body as she goes.

And despite the exotic sound of this adventure, it is no vacation. She is sick. She isn't Sherlock, observing the data with cool, calculating detachment. She *is* the data. Talking about yoga as a scientifically proven way to reduce stress is one thing, but actually doing yoga, in the throes of a devastating exhaustion syndrome and severe pain in the vulva, bladder, and sacral spines (for example) is really quite another. Unlike Peter, Susan, Edmund, and Lucy—and unlike Sherlock—she would like this adventure to be over.

But even so, it is hopeful work. Modern medicine has failed her, and she is going to do what it takes to heal her body, regardless of how it looks, regardless of what it takes.

She has, in essence, begun the journey of getting a Ph.D. in herself.

~

Now, as you know, I had already begun to dabble in alternative medicine.

And as any dabbler in alternatives can tell you, what begins as a serious endeavor can quickly devolve into all manner of woo. This is one of the major dangers of WOMI Narnia. Turkish delight is being hawked on just about every corner. Over the course of time, I may or may not have had crystals consecrated for each of my chakras, taken Native American mushrooms, tried every possible diet (vegan, raw, Ayurveda, paleo, macrobiotic, GAPS, SCD), and experimented with Chi Nei Tsang, craniosacral therapy, aromatherapy, osteopathy, Mayan uterine massage, EFT, shamans, ice baths, infrared saunas, binaural beats, self-hypnosis, and *The Secret*. I may or may not have tried to feng shui my colon back to health by moving my bookcase from the eastern to the southern wall.

But when I first came to San Francisco, I was absolutely focused. I was 100 percent determined to get better.

I had met the famous acupuncturist while she was visiting the East Coast, and as advertised, she was a miracle worker. Our first meeting and session were extraordinary. Like actual, real-life magic. It felt like white light itself had been unlocked in my cells, which threw off their wet, gray, scratchy cloaks—and this explosion of energy was more than enough to make me pack my bags and move across the country. What did I have to lose? Being chained to my childhood bed? I checked two suitcases and a guitar in the overhead. My mother helped me get on the plane, and my brother helped me once I got there. I intended to live cheaply in the basement of my aunt and uncle's house in San Francisco. I was not sure how it would all work out, or how I would take care of myself, but I decided to stay positive. On the airplane, I made lists on cocktail napkins of all the things I would do when I was healed.

Learn to cook.
Write songs.
Take a stage name—maybe Grandpa's name?
Make new friends.
Pray.
Do yoga.
Get a cat!
(Have sex.)

I was so hopeful.
I was so grateful.
I was the truest believer.

I had not even unpacked my suitcases before I hailed a taxi to take me over to the new acupuncturist's. I slept for three hours on the floor of the waiting room, and when it was finally my turn, she worked me over with a series of very quick, painful pinpricks. She assessed my overall health and balance of the five elements by feeling my pulses. She listened to the whole story, and told me that from a Chinese medicine perspective, I had a "profound lack of anger."

Gold star, I thought to myself. What a good girl.

The room was accented with Buddhist sculptures and exotic orchids. Holding my wrist, with eyes still closed, she prophesied that it would take six weeks to heal.

Six weeks!

My eyes watered, and my heart started to fill with joy.

If I had walked in feeling weak and wan and tired, I walked out feeling like Suzanne Somers.

~

Over the course of weeks and then months, I dutifully went to the acupuncturist, often many times a week. I also reunited with Alejandro del Sol, who was living in San Francisco, and hauled my exhausted, aching, barbed-wire self to his yoga class almost every day. I went back to a gut-healing paleo diet (I had veered into a vegetarian/Ayurvedic diet but now veered back), I meditated, visualized, detoxified, and dug deeply into my emotional life. I went to a Rolfer and a homeopath the acupuncturist recommended, I read loads of health and healing books, and I worked from home.

And noticeably, there was one central lesson everyone wanted to impart: this was my responsibility. One hundred percent. No one else could meditate for me, get to the appointments, change my diet, take the herbs, or stay positive at all costs.

Just me.

The time had come to take total responsibility for my life—and I accepted this, gladly.

Because regardless of how sick I still felt, or how much pain I was in, I was so grateful to have landed in this world, to have a dark yoga studio to go to, and a sacred practice, and a connection to my body. Ganesha smiled down, and I smiled back up. I learned to breathe, and stretch, slow down my mental chatter, control my mind, and relax. Finally.

For so many of us with bodies just barely connected to our heads, taking up yoga and self-care and finally sinking down into our neglected temples is the beginning of the way home.

~

This phase is best described as a WOMI's quiet and patient resuscitation of a broken spirit. It's almost impossible to move forward without it. It may sound a little hokey, but the truth is that any WOMI on this path needs to learn how to take care of her body— and also to begin caring for the Self. The soul. And as the ship starts to turn around on the voyage back to health, she can be sure that the inner voice will begin to make itself and its desires known. It wants to be heard. It has been locked away, thumping under the floorboards for too long.

So she might start to keep a journal, or take baths, or bring home flowers, or have dreams of significance. She will almost certainly begin to develop a relationship with the Universe, a modern stand-in for the divine.

She might start to think seriously about what she really wants out of life, and if she has not already, she might consider leaving her current soul-sucking job to do something a little more aligned. It is not an easy path to stay on, and the banshees will start to cry out—many of them in her own head, calling her selfish, silly, and stupid, and it can be a constant battle, reorienting herself from taking care of everything and everyone else—expectations, work, colleagues, family, partner, and children if she has them—to focusing on herself, her own heart, and her own body.

Caring for herself, she is a little surprised to learn, is a radical act.

~

I was shocked to see how poorly I had been taking care of myself, lo those twenty-nine years. I had grown up in a family where this kind of holistic behavior was associated with a sort of dim-wittedness, and I had always thought health nuts were just that—nuts. In my estimation, Count Chocula and Chef Boyardee had done a fine job keeping me fed and happy all my life. The way I strove to achieve, at just about everything, was a privilege—I would just as soon get off the success track to go chant and meditate as I would set fire to my many degrees. I would just as soon "buy organic" as I would buy the Brooklyn Bridge. I regularly got only about five hours of sleep—an indicator, I thought, of my strength—opting instead to study, work hard, and play hard. This is how I had been all my life, and it had suited me just fine.

It wasn't wild, self-destructive behavior.
In every way, I was exceedingly Standard.

But now that shit had monumentally hit the fan, I was beginning to see that my set point of normal—in the context of other cultures, and even compared to my own culture just a century ago—wasn't very normal at all. It was just normalized.

And, regardless of what I thought about all this in my mind, most of the basic woo things I was doing were really helping my body. I was in less pain. I had more energy. My skin cleared up. My digestion worked a little better. I was less afraid.

So I kept doing it.

I set up an altar, and a meditation space. I adopted a kitten from a shelter, and named her Mathilde. I began to do affirmations, and started to keep a journal. I made bone broth to sip morning and night. I prayed. It was a calm space in a painful, punishing storm. Having one sacred corner of life was a gift, and learning to be present helped move my mind away from the pain and onto small beauties I had never noticed before—the warmth of the running water, the smell of the rosemary at my gate, the brightness of my red kettle.

I knew how this sounded to others, so I was private about it. To the outside world, all this Stuart Smalley business sounds meaningless and ridiculous, but to the person who has been on the wrong end of a medical (or any other) battering ram for years, these practices are sustaining, necessary buttresses to an interior sense of self. The world may have become a giant echo chamber of pain and deaffirmation, and reinforcements are necessary.

From my new point of view, it was definitely better to be hokey than to drown in the sludge of my own cynicism.

And even though everything I had taken on was all-consuming—the acupuncture, the yoga, the self-care, the appointments, the food prep—I was beginning to feel empowered. My life felt like a slow-motion training montage.

I was beginning to feel in flashes that I was an agent in my own process—instead of at the mercy of a thousand machines and surgical masks—and now when the blows came hammering down (as they still did, often), I didn't have to roll over and just take it. My teachers wouldn't let me. They were intent on pushing me beyond what I thought I could do. They were very serious and did not indulge wallowing.

I loved this.

I was the Karate Kid.

And slowly, slowly, after a lot of waxing on and waxing off—it started to work.
Slowly, slowly, the miracle did start to unfold.
Slowly, slowly, I was brought back, again, partially, to the land of the living.

~

Now, it was not exactly a graceful spiral back to soaring health—it was a bumpy road, complicated just as much by doubting doctors as by shyster shamans. Along the way, I encountered as many quacks as my father warned me against when I started to veer away from the traditional path—my father, at that time, being the quintessential Western doctor, looking down on alternative medicine with great, pooh-poohing scorn—but I stuck to my guns and kept veering. I had finally found practitioners who took me seriously, and that base level of care was a foundation I could build on. I was starting to get measurably better for the first time since that blip in Maine in 2004. And for all the alternative quacks I encountered, the number was always equal to or less than the number of traditional hacks who had ever handed me a paper gown.

On this point of contrast, an example always sticks in my mind:

At the end of my time in New York, I'd met that woman I mentioned before, Charlotte, the secret twin, who had such a similar story to mine. And one of the key pieces to solving her puzzle had been getting treated for said controversial candidiasis. Even though I had gotten better from Diflucan so long ago, when I met Charlotte, I had not understood why. And so when she was telling me about it, it was the first time anyone had ever explained the all-over itching and the distended belly, the allergies, the brain fog, and the constant yeast infections. As she described my secret life back to me in living color, I wondered why, oh why, no one had ever mentioned this.

That's why I got significantly better on that medication my mother had prescribed. I'll be darned.

At Charlotte's recommendation, I had bought the alternative classic with the unfortunate jacket design, THE YEAST CONNECTION (caps not mine), and read it on the subway to class, which made for a wonderfully awkward commute to and from Columbia. But I could not put it down. I could not believe what I was reading. I wanted to start reciting it aloud to the people of the subway, and spread the good word. People get candida from overuse of antibiotics? Check. It colonizes the gut, which causes permeation in the lining, which makes you sensitive to everything? Check. You itch everywhere, especially your vagina, your eyes, and your rectum? Triple check. *Furry tongue?* I was ecstatic. All I had to do was stop eating sugar and alcohol (yeast feeds on sugar and alcohol) and take some antifungals.

I could not wait to treat my fungus.

"You know that's hocus-pocus, don't you?" chuckled a urologist, when I presented him with my candida discovery. "All those kooks are just taking people like you for a ride."

I was crestfallen.

But, but, I stammered, I'd already started treatment and was doing a little better. I knew this because I didn't have an itchy rectum anymore, which I considered a big, tangible step forward. I asked if it wasn't fair to measure success by how much my rectum did or did not itch?

He shrugged his shoulders.

I asked if he knew of another explanation for all of those weird symptoms?

Shrug.

He performed an excruciating manual exam.

I waddled out of the office that day with the number for a vaginal physical therapist in the Financial District, and a prescription for Elavil.

Elavil, of course, is an antidepressant.

6

I remember the exact moment I decided I was going to solve the mystery illnesses.

To be more specific, that I was going to (oh dear) "save women."

Not some of the women, but all of the women.

The year was 2009, and I was following up with the gastroenterologist who had first recommended Paxil a few years before—Paxil being the antidepressant that caused me to plummet from being upset-about-being-sick to being dangerously suicidal over the course of a few short months. But because of what I can only diagnose as pathological niceness, I did not bring this up at all in our follow-up conversation several years later. Water under the bridge, I thought. Be the bigger person, I thought. And also: Stay likable, so this well-respected doctor will continue to provide care on into the future.

Anyway, I wanted to speak with him about something completely different. I wanted to know what he could tell me about the helpful diet I had been eating and how it related to the evolving understanding of the science of the gut. While peristalsis was still an elusive factor for me, on my new grain- and sugar-free diet my distention had subsided, my digestion had improved, my food sensitivities had improved, and my energy had improved. I was hoping he could weigh in on the current research regarding gluten and sugar and probiotics—which had actually come a long way since my candida/hocus-pocus meeting about three years before. I had read plenty of shiny diet books that glossed these things in general terms, but they tended to be light on real science—and I wanted to hear from Real Science. I thought my doctor could help me stay on the straight and narrow, and guard against my being taken in by any of the various dietary fads and factions. Because, you see, I had—and I continue to have—a deep and abiding respect for physicians. I respect how intelligent they are, how rigorously educated, and I respect how dedicated they are to helping other people. I grew up in a warren of doctors, and so I do know how hard the job is.

However, when I brought these earnest dietary questions to Dr. Paxil, he could not suppress a loud snort.

"Sarah," he said with a sigh. "Please eat whatever you want. You have irritable bowel syndrome, and food has nothing to do with irritable bowel syndrome."

And I remember that time seemed to slow for just a moment.

This claim, *food has nothing to do with the organ that processes food*, seemed almost cartoonishly disconnected from logic and reason.

But there he was, saying it as if he were saying the sky was blue.

And for a passing moment, it felt like I was in the 1960s, with a lung condition, looking across the desk at my pulmonologist, who was looking back at me, blithely smoking a cigarette.

I felt a muscle of righteousness, deep within, starting to twitch.

"Did you know fifty-one percent of women complain of constipation?" he asked. "It's true—so what I like to tell women like you is that you're actually quite *normal*."

He was smiling. He was genuinely trying to make me feel better. I was smiling, too. I was genuinely thinking:

You sent the wrong girl down the rabbit hole.

~

I leapt into researching these subjects with a verve not commonly associated with chronic fatigue syndrome.

I went *full* Hermione, with stacks of books, walls of index cards and articles, and reams of studies piled high around me, deeply immersing myself in the science and research of things like diet, sleep, meditation, and yoga. Because I was truly unsettled that so many people around me were obviously getting at least somewhat better by adopting these healthy behaviors—yet their doctors still wrote "Spontaneous remission" in their charts when they reported their improvements, waving away the details, snorting all the way.

This just couldn't be right.
And, of course, it wasn't.

When I did just the minutest amount of research into the basics of the alternative health movement—eating real food, moving your body, sleeping enough, using fewer endocrine-disrupting products, getting enough social connection—it did not take very long to conclude that alternative medicine's best asset in the medical cold war between East and West was actually, surprisingly:

The Data.

When it came to the importance of those basic ideas, it turned out they weren't very "alternative" at all. And because of this, there really was a lot of cold, hard data. Which was thrilling. Because as any health journeyer can tell you, when things threaten to get impossibly woo, fringe, or all caps—cold, hard data is a real blessing.

And so I swan-dove into JSTOR, PubMed, *JAMA,* and *The New England Journal of Medicine,* drinking it all in, knowing that I was fortifying myself for my newly conceived woman-saving quest. Because the basic conclusion was pretty clear. If you focused on what all the different health fads and factions had in common, and ignored their fringier claims—you found the same recommendations over and over again. Eat real food, don't use too many problematic chemicals, sleep enough, move enough, relax enough, repeat. And for these central claims, you didn't have to cherry-pick your studies—when it came to the basics of health, there was an entire cherry *orchard* of data waiting—hulking, gigantic, and wondering where everyone has been.

Indeed, I started to see that the frothed, religious debate in the health circles people were always trying to get me to join—paleo versus vegan, CrossFit versus yoga, West versus East, gluten-as-myth versus gluten-as-Satan, and so on—was detracting from the basics of the health movement, and repelling the medical men and women of logic and reason.

And this went to the heart of the problem.

I wasn't wrong to want a credible source to help keep me on the straight and narrow. But I wasn't going to get that from a Dr. Paxil or a Dr. Hocus-Pocus. Because as I sat there researching in 2009, it was very clear that the *basics* of the health movement were not accepted or integrated as scientifically meaningful in the regular medical community. Certainly not as meaningful as medication, surgery, or 3-D printers. Except for thirty seconds of mechanical lip service about eating less and exercising more, there just was not an easily accessible, credible, white-coated source to help keep you on the straight and narrow.

That was the problem.

That basic foundation of how to create health was just missing. It was simply not there.
It was not part of the training, and therefore it was never going to be a meaningful part of the treatment plan—for me or for anyone else.

And just to reiterate: I could *completely understand why*. I was a normal person once. I was one of those people who routinely threw things like diet change, sleep, acupuncture, and yoga under the bus as placebo nincompoopery, superstition, preening, or naïveté—and this was easy to do before I became sick. Before I got sick, I would say the same things many of my doctors were saying to me now, and with the same condescension: "The data is not in!" "Show me the data!" Even though I had no idea if the data was in or not. For understandable (and frankly delicious) reasons, I and pretty much everyone else I knew was hoping upon hope that Science would do us a solid, prove all those woo-woo zealots wrong, and leave us to our Twizzlers, Lucky Charms, and stuffed-crust pizzas.

But unfortunately for us standard Americans, of whom I was definitely one for about twenty-six years, we were wrong.

The research was clear.

How we ate, slept, thought, and moved—these things really mattered, in a foundational way.
Pooh-poohing them was no longer scientifically sound.

In other words, I was delighted to learn that my best asset so far was actually, surprisingly:

The Data.

~

Now, this turn as private eye will be familiar to the common WOMI. As a group, we really are a very studious bunch, but I think the reasons are pretty straightforward.

If we take chronic fatigue syndrome as an example, we find that these patients almost uniformly describe their chief symptoms as something akin to having the flu, just turned down a notch or two.
That is, an ever so slightly tamed flu.
Flu Junior.

And here is the thing:

When you have Flu Junior—but unlike Flu Senior, it never, ever goes away—you simply don't have the option to ignore it. Or to accept it as the new normal. Or to try to antidepress your way out of it. It just doesn't matter how stoic or positive you think you are—no one can accept 75 percent, 50 percent, or even 25 percent of a mysterious, permanent flu. No one. Not anyone. Not a young person, not an old person. Not a man, not a woman. Not in a plane, not on a train. No matter who you are, if you have any percentage of the flu, you must—must—seek help.

Which works quite well when people want to help you. And quite poorly when they don't.

And as you are acutely aware by now, in this case they don't. And this leads people like me to a pretty uniform conclusion.

If no one is going to help you solve the mystery: You've just got to solve it for yourself.

~

Thus, I continued to dig deeper and deeper into the issues at hand. Down and down I went, and once I was firmly ensconced in the briars and brambles, there slowly but surely began to emerge from the texts another looming and indisputable member of that-which-was-no-longer-up-for-debate. While I was still an advocate for the health basics, a new topic soon began to eclipse all else, swiftly becoming my focus, my favorite, my precious. It was fascinating, and complicated, and relevant, and weird, and this topic was:

The gut.
The modern, over-antibioticed, standard American dieted, leaky, dysbiotic gut.

"The road to health is paved with good intestines" went the common saying in my research, and as I dug and dug, I knew that this was true. Not hundreds, but thousands of studies suggested this was true. Yet at the time, even in 2009, this was still a very novel idea.

Soon my world would revolve almost entirely around this discovery. Because once you moved past the more general healthy behaviors—and their association with generally feeling better—and started to really get down to the question of what was *specifically* causing autoimmunity, fibromyalgia, and chronic fatigue syndrome, if one thing seemed to bind together all the myriad symptoms of the mysteriously ill, it definitely appeared to be our dysbiotic, leaky guts.

So what is a dysbiotic, leaky gut?

I thought you would never ask.

Dysbiosis.
dys.bio.sis | dis ˈbīo sis| noun
An imbalance in the microflora of the intestines; a shift of the ratio of beneficial bacteria to pathogenic bacteria.

In the human body we have an almost unsettling number of guests—bacteria, fungi, viruses, and other microbes. So many, in fact, that one could even start to think that it's actually we humans who are the guests—there is at least a 1:1 ratio of microbial cells to human cells in any individual, and by some estimates even more.

A gloriously creepy idea.

As a whole, this inner ecosystem is now famously known as the microbiome. There are several small biomes throughout the body—in the eyes, ears, mouth, nose, skin, vagina—but the biggest biome by far is in the gut. It weighs in at about three pounds, and consists of roughly *100 trillion cells*. For reference, the human brain also weighs three pounds, and 100 trillion cells outnumber all the stars in our galaxy—many times over.

The microbiome is a big deal.

And until the last decade, the research on the benefits of the microbiome were comparatively spare, flying beneath the radar of most physicians—with the emphasis on microbes previously being that they are the bad guys, and need to be killed off. This turns out to be partially, and maybe mostly, wrong. Mostly, we need our microbes, and we are only now beginning to understand what a vastly important, if silent, role they play at every level of health. And so *dysbiosis* is simply a term for when that inner ecosystem becomes imbalanced. We have up to one thousand species living in the gut, and, as with any ecosystem in the wild, there is a natural balance of flora and fauna—and if you remove certain important species, especially very quickly, you will begin to observe all kinds of ecological disruptions and potential problems. All ecologies have a natural balance, and each species has its function in relation to the rest.

What researchers are looking at now—and it is widely felt that this will be one of the most important areas of medical study in the twenty-first century—is the purpose, function, and dysfunction of the microbiome. And they have already identified many, many, many links between a host of diseases and adverse consequences that result from knocking our invisible guests so far out of their natural balance.

So how did we do that?

Well, it will come as no surprise that our diet plays a prominent, significant role. The mechanisms are not totally clear, but it has been shown in animal models that a high-sugar, low-fiber, low-ferment diet promotes the overgrowth of "bad" bacteria, and inhibits the proliferation of "good" bacteria.

But then, unfortunately, the other major problem when it comes to dysbiosis very much seems to be our lifesaving arsenal of antibiotics. It has been repeatedly shown that the chronic use of broad-spectrum antibiotics is one of the drivers behind dysbiosis—which is really too bad, considering how great antibiotics are. It creates a bit of a conundrum—much like the conundrum of the expedient, delicious, cheap, but ultimately unhealthy American diet.

Antibiotics were first put to widespread use to combat previously fatal infections in the 1940s—a quantum leap that completely revolutionized the practice of medicine, inaugurated the age of the miracle pill, and continues to save countless lives, every day, every hour, every minute. Antibiotics rightly deserve a standing ovation from the world for all but eradicating some of the worst plagues known to man.

But this good work does not inoculate the miracle pills from being able to cause their own problems. It is now well known that overusing antibiotics can cause resistant strains of bacteria to develop (like MRSA), and what researchers are only just starting to understand is that the overuse of antibiotics can disrupt our delicate inner ecology, permanently decimating certain species, and leaving the ecosystem unable to do what it did so perfectly, and so quietly, before.

This is all relatively new to Western medicine, but it is not a new idea in alternative circles. More and more practitioners have come around to the idea that, just as Chinese medicine posits, the gut is the seat of health, "the Mother," and is responsible for nourishing the whole of the body. And science bears this out. We now know that our microbes are responsible for training our immune system, that our "good" microbes can be considered *part* of our immune system, and that they fight against and keep out pathogenic bacteria. They also digest certain foods and fibers, they produce specific vitamins (like vitamin K) and short-chain fatty acids (like butyrate) that are essential for health, and they can even switch some of our genes on and off. And this is just the tip of the iceberg.

The takeaway is:
We need our bugs.

When we clear-cut this forest, it doesn't always grow back the way it was—especially in certain types of individuals. Instead, we know that after the deforestation, and especially in the presence of a poor diet, pathogenic microbes have the opportunity to overgrow and take over the jungle. The level of overgrowth will differ from person to person, depending on a variety of factors, including which type of antibiotic was used, previous antibiotic usage, diet, etc. These overgrowths of pathogenic microbes include, but are not limited to, *Clostridium difficile, Klebsiella,* and our favorite, verboten, phantom fungus: *Candida albicans.*

But back in 2007, 2008, 2009, these ideas were more of a rumbling, not an accepted, if daunting, theory. And most of the first rumblers were alternative and integrative practitioners.

Still, I was sure they were rumbling the right tune—largely because the idea resonated like a big, fat tuning fork in my own story.

I had become inexplicably ill—for reasons that were not understood—but the fallout of which was almost textbook Modern Gut Problems from an alternative medicine perspective. To save my life, I had been given an enormous, *enormous* amount of antibiotics, and was even sent back to school with an IV PICC line in my arm—for a month—which was all, of course, for my safety. I was lucky to be alive, and if I had become septic in an age before antibiotics, I likely would have died.

But again, saving a life is not always without consequence. As I developed more and more problems—yeast infections, thrush (a yeast infection of the mouth), severe bowel problems, severe fatigue, severe aching, allergies, and severe brain fog—it all remained a mystery. My stool was even tested to make sure I didn't have anything clinically serious, and we were told I didn't.

The trouble is, the tests that are used in conventional medicine are only calibrated to pick up acute infections. These imbalances of good flora and bad flora are considered "subclinical" and do not register on a normal stool test, because a basic imbalance is not life-threatening. Beyond those two black and white poles—acute infection or nothing—everything else is considered irrelevant. (And, have I mentioned, physicians are usually some shade of hostile to hearing about the importance of these suspected "imbalances"?)

The trouble is, that opinion and/or hostility are becoming less and less scientifically sound.

And the most troubling trouble is, there is a much more important reason to take dysbiosis seriously, other than jeopardizing your digestive/nutrient/genetic and immune status (as if disrupting those is not already scary enough).

It is now thought that a simple, untreated imbalance of micro-flora can lead to a low-grade, long-term inflammation in the intestinal epithelium (the inner lining of the gut)—and it is thought that this long-term, low-grade inflammation can lead directly to the phenomenon now known, augustly, as:

Leaky gut syndrome.
leak.y gut syn.drome | ˈlēkē gət ˈsin͵drōm| noun
The loosening of the tight junctions in the epithelial lining of the gut, which may allow food particles, toxins, and bacterial waste into the bloodstream.

Leaky gut is also known as increased intestinal permeability (IIP), or intestinal hyperpermeability, and in contrast to the widespread medical opinion that it doesn't exist, or is an Internet fad—it is the opposite of a fringe, understudied phenomenon. There are over ten thousand academic papers detailing the causes, the associated diseases, and the possible treatments for increased intestinal permeability.

Leaky gut syndrome is just what it sounds like—a gut that is more permeable than it should be. Normally, our food is broken down into tiny particles in the intestine and then absorbed through the microvilli into the bloodstream. A common description of the microvilli lining the gut wall is that it's like shag carpeting. In between each shag, there is a junction that can be opened and closed to let nutrients through, but the junction generally stays closed to keep most things contained. But when the lining of the gut is breached—that is, the junctions between those microvilli are widened, going from regular panty hose to fishnet stockings—then all manner of nontiny food particles, toxins, and bacterial wastes are allowed to start seeping into the bloodstream. These things would normally have been kept relatively safe in the intestinal tract, as the epithelial lining of the gut is much like the epithelial lining of the skin: there to keep most stuff out. But when food is allowed into the blood partially undigested, those particles are no longer either nutritious or innocuous. In the bloodstream, undigested, they become:

Antigens.

an.ti.gens | ˈantijəns| noun

Toxins or other foreign substances that induce an immune response in the body, esp. the production of antibodies.

Antigen, as the author of *The Autoimmune Epidemic*, Donna Nakazawa, says, is one of the most important words of the twenty-first century.

Antigens activate the immune system. They may not cause symptoms at all, at least not at first, and our bodies are constantly policing for these kinds of things, flagging them, and removing them without our knowing. But as you can imagine, if this red flag is going up all day, every day—then you are going to have one highly activated immune system.

And it is this breached intestinal wall, and subsequent near-constant activation of the immune system—that is, a new, modern state of antigen overload due largely to dysbiosis and the attendant leaky gut—which is now theorized (with more and more data to support the theory) to be one of the major sources of a previously mysterious problem I may have mentioned here and there:

Autoimmune disease.

As we remember, an autoimmune disease is when the body mistakes its own tissue for a foreign invader and starts to attack itself. It has long been thought that this error might occur because the body starts to mistake itself for different antigens—called "molecular mimicry," when an antigen is molecularly similar to a protein or tissue in the body—but it was not clear why it would make this mistake in the first place, or why so many more bodies seem to be making this mistake over the last thirty years that autoimmunity has started to skyrocket.

But in the context of a new, major, modern problem—that is, the tremendous uptick in the chronic overuse of antibiotics, which can lead to a breach in the gut and then to a bloodstream flooded with antigens, perhaps consistently and for a very long time—that mistake makes significantly more sense.

If someone were setting off my alarm system all day, every day, I just assume it would break down.

So following this new, important information that is at the forefront of scientific study at the moment, one may or may not be surprised to learn both a leaky gut and a high flow of antigenic material have been correlated in the literature with a few other syndromes. Namely:

Fibromyalgia.
Sick building syndrome.
Post-treatment Lyme disease syndrome.
Chronic fatigue syndrome.

Just this once, I will cherry-pick a study for you:
At Cedars-Sinai Medical Center, they did a study to test for small intestinal bacterial overgrowth (SIBO) in forty-two test subjects with fibromyalgia. Considering that the cause of fibromyalgia is unknown, totally mysterious, and very difficult to treat, any correlation at all, even 30 percent of patients, would have been interesting and encouraging.

So how many of the forty-two patients with fibromyalgia had SIBO?
Forty-two.
I'm no scientist, but 100 percent is a pretty compelling metric.

In fact, in those ten thousand papers mentioned earlier, leaky gut and an antigenic flow are also correlated with many types of immune dysregulation, such as allergies, food sensitivities, mast cell activation syndrome, mold illness, skin conditions, and asthma. Which, to your narrator and researcher, seemed (and still seems) deeply, profoundly, amazingly, wonderfully:

Relevant.

A big, fat, hulking common denominator.

And, *and* if all of that were not enough—if we go back to the science of what exactly is triggering the loosening of the tight junctions, because they don't just do it spontaneously—the pioneer of this entire theory, Dr. Alessio Fasano, a professor at Harvard Medical School, explains that his big discovery was that the gut junctions are not actually forced open, or punctured—they are mediated and controlled by the release of a protein called *zonulin*. (Another *Mork & Mindy* component to our working theory.) When zonulin is released, the tight junctions between the microvilli widen.

And of the known triggers for the release of the protein zonulin, there are two that stand out in the research as consistently more common than all the rest.

You, educated reader, now know one of the main ones:

Dysbiosis, or a long-term imbalance of the gut flora.

And would the reader like to know the other?

It's gluten.

The protein found in wheat, gliadin, has been clearly demonstrated to trigger the release of the leaky gut–inducing protein, zonulin. This elevated level of zonulin is found in most celiac patients—but it is *also* found in many patients with chronic illness, on ingesting gluten. This phenomenon is called non-celiac gluten sensitivity, or NCGS. These people have been shown to also have leaky guts, high levels of zonulin, reactivity to gliadin passing into the bloodstream, and, unsurprisingly, all the usual mysterious symptoms, miseries, and illnesses. Hence the ubiquity of miracle healings once patients remove just gluten from their diet, even in the absence of celiac disease.

Thank you, Dr. Fasano.

Things are starting to make a lot more sense.

~

Now, none of this is to say the human gut and its myriad modern problems are all mapped out and a dream to treat—not at all. Nor are dysbiosis and gluten the only triggers for leaky gut—not at all. In fact, the next class of common triggers should not be a surprise, since we're so familiar with the basics of health. The next class of material that promotes a leaking gut are certain chemicals and pesticides. Also NSAIDs and birth-control pills. That is, the unfortunate reality is that we live in a highly antigenic, highly zonulinic world. Furthermore, a leaking gut is not the only way antigens get into the bloodstream—we absorb chemicals in our skin, use them in most of our beauty products, breathe them in, and absorb them simply by ingesting them, for example, in foods covered in pesticides—and all of this is thought to likewise play a role in overactivating the immune system (among other negative effects), which may eventually lead to the immune dysregulation associated with autoimmune disease and many of the other mysterious illnesses.

That said, it does appear that the gut seems to be the overwhelming source of the antigenic flow, and this is important to know as a jumping-off point—that is, reducing dangerous chemicals in the home, in the majority of people with these problems, would be secondary to focusing seriously on the state of their intestine: its barrier, its flora, and its overall state of function.

Even so, it's important to understand that these illnesses result from an aggregate of all of these factors. As I was coming to learn, deep in the weeds of PubMed, the microbiome *itself*—and the many modern problems associated with it—actually may provide a useful parallel to a mysterious illness.

It is complex.
It is multifactorial.
And to heal, it requires the most daunting thing of all: personal change.

In my now-yearlong inquiry, it was becoming very clear to me that some fundamental, adverse changes had been made to the foundations of our health over the last century—particularly to our microbiome, to our diet, to our environment—that were not perfectly understood yet, but clearly required some kind of fundamental, foundational response. Both from the patient, and from the physician. And that meant that what we were really seeking was not a simple tweak, or supplement, or new medication alone. What we were really in need of was an entire paradigm shift. Which was unfortunate. Because no one likes an entire paradigm shift.

But that didn't matter to me.
Because I am a woman of logic and reason.

While once there was a time when no one knew any of this gut stuff, nutrition stuff, toxin stuff, lifestyle stuff—that time was coming to an end.

Enough data was in.
At least enough to be paying serious attention.

As I would soon start to preach from high atop my box of soap:
In this modern world, with these modern illnesses, it was now critically, *critically,* important for a WOMI to find a physician or practitioner who was up-to-date on this literature, and who would take her diet and her biome into account.

And really, for the simplest of simple reasons.
It was the scientific thing to do.

7

Back at the ranch, as pleased as I was with my gradual physical progress—and as pleased as I was with my new, slightly more cerebral understanding of what was going on—it was also starting to become clear to me that my healing plan was still missing one critical element. I had taken responsibility, I had learned diaphragmatic breathing, I had mastered Warrior Pose—just as I had changed my diet, reinvented my personal product regimen, and made sure I was getting enough deep sleep . . . but even so, there was still one glaring deficiency in my life, and it was the famous, ancient supersupplement known as:

People.

WOMIs can have a very difficult time with People, and this makes sense. Illness is extremely isolating. Language and communication are big issues for us (not having a proper name is a much bigger deal than you might think), and shame is a big issue for us (ours are not considered the noble ailments of the lionhearted, but the nagging, embarrassing concerns of the oversensitive). Pelvic pain does not imbue a young woman with a particularly buoyant sense of personal esteem, and the same can be said for a urologic disease, a bowel disease, a thyroid condition, or possession by an invisible lethargy monster. And so even though the problem may be crippling, devastating, or humiliating, there is no pamphlet to hand out that can help create a space of understanding.

The inverse of Harry Potter, the mysteriously ill are dearly in need of an anti-invisibility cloak.

After six years of being sick, I *still* hadn't told almost anyone what was going on. Which, in retrospect, is hard to fathom. I have a lot of friends, and a big family, and we all love one another, a lot. But I just could not, would not, let go of the hope that it would just somehow all get better and I could go back to normal, without ever having to say anything to anyone about my vagina.

But that attitude, in addition to the limiting factors of my illness, had caused me to grow further and further apart from all of them. The daily colonoscopy preps (which I had come to call the "Bowel Olympics") kept me in my bathroom much of the day. I didn't have the energy to do much of anything besides yoga and taking care of my basic needs. But most important, when I did try to explain what was going on with me, there was too much darkness, and too many personal details—and I had honestly been stung too many times by the barbs of disbelief, even from my close friends. So over time, I had just stopped returning people's calls. And as any WOMI knows, this is one of the most painful paradoxes. You are at a time in your life when you need friends more than ever, but are missing the lexicon to communicate your distress and your needs.

However, I had been lapsing in and out of this isolation shameber for six years now, and it was just too painful to keep up for much longer. I finally decided that the only way to be understood was to make myself understood—and two days before Christmas of that year, I stayed up all night and wrote an epic, colo-vago-centric e-mail for all of my people—friends, family, campaign coworkers— explaining everything, every last thing, no gruesome holds barred. I explained why I had disappeared into the ether, and explained how hard it was to connect. I explained the Bowel Olympics and my extremely low reserves of energy. I also explained to the best of my knowledge what was wrong, explained what I was doing to get better, and explained how challenging it was to be met with a wall of skepticism from those I loved.

I was terrified to press Send.

But I did, and by morning, an enormous outpouring of support had come flooding in—aunts, uncles, college friends, childhood friends, and friends of friends. People thanked me for explaining things, explaining my disappearance, and explaining what would be helpful going forward. And most important, they all acknowledged this did, in fact, really suck. And that it was serious.

And oh, for a moment, I did feel valid again.

I had been Seen, and a huge weight began to lift from my shoulders. In one simple act of witness and self-witness, it was truly the best Christmas gift I had ever received.

It gave me strength.

I had worn a deep groove into the road to my acupuncturist's office, the road to the yoga studio down the street, and the road to the neighborhood grocery store. Beyond that, the world was too wild, too woolly. Everyone else in California seemed to me a choir of strangers, a thousand voices deep, booming *But You Look! Just! Fine!*

And yet, something had to be done.

I remember this very well—it was a cold Monday night in February and Valentine's Day had just come and gone, in the most depressing way. Despite the slow, upward spiraling I was experiencing in my body, I was still spending most of my time with my cat (Mathilde), my sheep-shaped hot-water bottle, my starfish-shaped ice pack, and the *Twilight* series.

I couldn't take it anymore. I pulled my dormant guitar from the closet, and got in the car.

~

The famous San Francisco open mic at the Hotel Utah is not a normal open mic. Normal open mics are generally an anemic affair—seven or eight locals singing Bob Dylan covers to a restaurant crowd that isn't listening.

Not at the Hotel Utah.

Unbeknownst to me when I headed over, up to eighty people often sign up to play every Monday night, some of them the best of the local San Francisco music scene, while at least fifty more come to watch. The Utah is an institution—an old saloon, built in 1908, with dark wood, twinkling lights, and a full bar, which is put to good use.

So when I pushed the door open, I ran straight into a wall of well-liquored singers, comedians, drummers, bass players, banjo players, fiddlers, and classical pianists. I froze. I had never played to a crowd that big by myself—I actually barely knew how to play the guitar. My heart started jumping out of my chest, and my intestines twisted their barbed wire around their cemented content. I'm not up for this, I thought—suddenly wishing for the dark yoga studio, the orchids, Alejandro, Ganesha—and just as my nerves were about to get the best of me, they suddenly, divinely, gave me diarrhea instead. For someone with almost zero independent intestinal motility, it was like a peristaltic act of God. Never in the history of nice young women has someone been so relieved to get the runs. I emerged from the bathroom absolutely radiant and I signed up just before the name drawing began, slipping into a dark corner to wait for my number. "Wolf Larsen, you're number twenty," said the host. Twenty was a very good number to get, and Wolf Larsen was my Nebraskan grandfather's name—an alias I had dreamed up months before on a JetBlue Airways cocktail napkin.

~

In the alternative medicine world, following your bliss is highly correlated to healing. Story after story crops up of the woman who left her corporate job to work with wild horses, or to become a painter, or a kindergarten teacher, or a health coach—magically eliminating all of her ailments, and giving her a whole new lease on life. Often this is called "the gift of illness."

I knew this, and thought it sounded like the most excellent solution to my problems yet. Do what you love to do and Be Healed?

Yes, please.

From that night on, I was a Monday-night regular at the Utah.

I made friends, I found a warm, supportive, eccentric family of musicians, and everyone thought my name really was Wolf. I was fairly open with them from the beginning about my illness. And despite continued, searing vaginal and spinal pain, I was beginning to feel happy again. Music and community were incredible vitamins. I was terribly ill during the day with the pain and the pooping and the aching and the exhaustion—but once that was more or less over, which for me was nighttime, I was free to go to the ball. I could only do something like that once a week, but for me once a week was a huge step forward. I was leaving the house.

And soon, I was playing occasional gigs around the city. I started writing music in my little studio apartment, prolifically. Wolf Larsen was on the radio. Wolf Larsen had fans and a following. Now when I walked down the street in the Mission, people sometimes said, "Hey, Wolf," and I would nod, keep walking, and start grinning from ear to ear.

It was all very exciting, but most important: I was really starting to get better.

Everyone noticed it.

8

That was a lovely year.

I was playing music.
I was staying out later and later.
I was making friends.
I was starting to have the odd whiskey now and then.
I was flirting.

Because it was fun.
Because I could.

And at home, I was researching up a storm.
My apartment looked like the national archive for bacterial data.
I was beginning to interview WOMIs left and right.

I was solving mysteries.
In fact:
I was starting to write a book.
This book.
A woman-saving book.

I was so excited about it.

I was starting to have a vision for how this nightmare story might all end, and it was looking very good.

And then?

And then, after all that time, and all those years, and all that wandering—after all that WOMI-this and WOMI-that—one day, what I had been searching and searching and searching for was delivered, quite unexpectedly, right to my front door.

One day, a day like any other day, I woke to find that I was suddenly the owner of:

A Diagnosis.

9

While it was indeed a lovely year (comparatively speaking), it was also true that toward the end of those twelve months my improvement began to plateau. I was enjoying the life I had painstakingly put back together, but it was hard not to notice that I still had to receive acupuncture two to three times a *week* just to keep myself from going down the drain—which is a lot of acupuncture, and a lot of dollars. I was grateful for my gradual improvement—deeply grateful—but the amount of care I required was unsustainable. The motors in my cells were starting to run again, my muscles ached only some of the time, and my hope machines were firing on all cylinders—but the bear trap on my pelvic nerves was still snug as ever, and the gut remained twenty-two feet of flaccid cement. Those were just the facts. No matter how much yoga I did—and I had developed some serious tone in my previously wobbly appendages—I still had severe spinal, abdominal, ovarian, vaginal, and bladder pain, which was actually getting worse. Yoga helped me in nearly every way, with one important exception: it seemed to exacerbate the nerve pain. And this was difficult to say aloud in a quiet class of yogi seekers, especially considering where the nerve pain was. Alejandro would come over to push my pelvis deeper into the ground during Upward Dog, which would elicit an earsplitting yelp, which would elicit a disapproving look from the master. I tried to explain the problem, but he encouraged me to stay strong and keep pushing. Mind over matter, he told me.

The problem was that everyone had been saying this for almost two years. Just keep pushing. Keep fighting, Warrior. I was grateful for my improvement, but the reality was that the work and the cost of care required just to stay functional was not possible to keep up over the long term—it was my full-time job, except I was paying someone else to keep this job—and I was no longer trending upward. What we were doing was not getting to the root of the problem, and I had done everything I was asked. I had driven myself to all the appointments, walked myself to the studio, pushed through the exhaustion, stretched through the pain, changed in every way I was asked to change, cultivated my inner smile, and affirmed myself to high heaven.

I really, really did not want to rock the warm, happy boat I had been sailing in—but it still felt like the barbed, iron claw of doom was reaching up through my vagina, intent on slowly crushing my bladder and intestines. And I guess I don't know very many people who can make peace with a barbed, iron claw of vaginal doom.

So I rocked the happy boat.

In a fit of uncharacteristic anger, directed at all of these very nice people, I called each practitioner up, one by one, and I demanded a collective rethinking of my disease. I think I might have even yelled, and I'm no yeller.

Oh, I felt so embarrassed, and so ashamed. I was yelling at an acupuncturist. I had spent all this time learning how to practice gratitude and loving kindness, and here I was doing what I had learned was the worst thing of all—letting my emotions get the best of me. But something was still wrong, and a deeper part of me that didn't care about affirmations and positivity continued to rage.

And to my enormous frustration, the acupuncturist was not put off at all. She was happy to see me so feisty. She said when the anger finally surfaces, the patient is about to have a breakthrough.

And in a way, she was right.

~

My fit precipitated a series of appointments with traditional Western doctors again, which immediately precipitated a visit from my mother. My left labia had become so swollen that it stuck outside the vagina, for which they said I could try a labiaplasty. But they also said the swelling would probably find another outlet even if we removed the labia. Then my bowel function was still so bad that they said I could just do a bowel resection and live with an ostomy bag. But they also said that might make the abdominal pain worse, and it was up to me whether or not I wanted to risk life with a bag in addition to more pain.

I was not enjoying life outside the warm, happy boat.

But in the middle of all this, my mother was upstairs with my aunt and uncle, faxing my records to a new gynecologist, when she looked down, and happened to notice a blip in one of the old GI lab reports. It read, "Negative, Negative, Negative, No Specimen, Negative." And my mother, top-notch doctor that she is, knew that "No Specimen" did not mean, "Negative."

She called the lab.

"No Specimen," they said, would mean that the test was ordered, but never performed. No sample was ever sent in from the doctor, back in 2003. The missing test was for a parasite called *Strongyloides,* a roundworm, a tropical parasite. Doctor Mom went on the Internet to just see if it would be plausible to retest me for the disease. The Internet informed her that *Strongyloides* can cause:

Paralysis of the bowel.
Searing abdominal pain.
Itching in the rectum and ears.
Coinfections and fungal overgrowth.
Fatigue.
Myalgic aching in the muscles and bones.
Distention of the stomach.
Organ failure and death.

My doctor mother dragged me to the lab and ordered the blood work herself.

Two days later, I found her on my doorstep, buzzing and buzzing and buzzing the buzzer.

"Positive," she said, sobbing. "Off the charts positive."

~

Long story short, it turned out I had a very real case of *Strongyloides stercoralis,* a roundworm I probably picked up as a teenager in Costa Rica. The worms can lay dormant for years, until unleashed by a triggering event.

We quickly learned that chronic strongyloidiasis can initiate or mimic an autoimmune disease, can paralyze the bowel, can crowd out beneficial bacteria, and can pave the way for an overgrowth of pathogenic bacteria and fungi, or dysbiosis. And unlike regular dysbiosis, *Strongyloides* worms absolutely have to be treated with strong medication. *Strongyloides* worms can also feed on nerve endings wherever they are concentrated most—with rare cases reported in the urinary and gynecologic systems—which causes burning, excruciating pain. The mortality rate for an untreated hyperinfective syndrome is 90 percent.

We called several of the doctors who had been working on my unsolved case for so many years—all top-notch physicians—to get their opinions on this discovery, and the response was universally the same.

"Holy fucking shit."

~

That was my response, too.

It really felt like I had been handed the perfect setup for an end to this long nightmare. A divine alley-oop for the microbial manifesto I had been preparing on my soapbox, not to mention hard proof that it was not all in my pretty little head. The Universe had spoken.

What I had been researching and learning, I was now going to nail to the wall, and prove the theory by getting better myself.

I was Michael Jordan, sailing toward the net.

In the next chapter of my life—with my divine diagnosis and scientific vindication—I was going to be on the royal road to health.

In the long argument over my body, I was going to Win.

Reader, it pains me to think about the next chapter of my life.

In the days following Revelation, I pulled out a sheaf of paper.

"Dear Dr. X: You may not remember me, but I remember you."

I went on to explain to several of the more unpleasant doctors I had seen over the years the nuances of a *Strongyloides* infection, as well as an armchair analysis of leaky gut syndrome, coinfections, and the connection to the mysterious illnesses. As a service to them (so they could better understand patients like me in the future), the letter served as a recap of the many blind alleys, misdiagnoses, and red herrings we had all seen along my complicated eight-year medical journey—culminating in my final missed diagnosis of a tropical illness, Watson.

I attempted to refrain from finger wagging, but in the end a strong overtone of nanny-nanny-boo-boo could not be helped.

When I was diagnosed with that gnarly intestinal infection, with the attendant bowel flora catastrophe and its miasma of associated symptoms—leaky gut, inflammation, food sensitivities, allergies, fatigue, pain—I could not have felt more vindicated. Exactly as I had been whistle-blowing for some time, the seat of the Problem was in the gut. It was in my gut, and everyone's guts. Guts were the answer. And indeed, articles confirming my wild ideas were starting to pour into the mainstream—a big article in *The New Yorker* about the microbiome, a big article in *The New York Times* about fecal transplants (my in-box continues to overflow with forwards from friends every time an article comes out about fecal transplants), a book called *Gulp,* by the wonderful Mary Roach, about the importance of the digestive tract. NPR's *Radiolab* aired an excellent series of shows dedicated to parasites, the gut, autoimmune disease, and intestinal permeability.

Sweet, sweet victory.

And as for my own situation, now that we had something to focus all of our energy on, I felt very sure that my life was now free to proceed the way I was told the health journey is meant to proceed—healthy living, healthy loving, and following my bliss. Once I just eliminated the bad actor in my body and healed up my gut, I could get back to the business of being a normal twenty-nine-year-old. I could, for example, leave the house anytime I wanted. I could, for another example, think about having an epic romance. Or I could think about starting a family. Or I could finally start building a career—possibly raising awareness around the gathering storm of autoimmune disease, and sounding the alarm about our collective intestinal problem, and making over women's health as a matter of general public concern, as opposed to the sole interest of OB-GYN doctors, belittled for their pink scrubs.

All great ideas.

There was just one problem.

And it was the same problem as always.

Just like in the emergency room, when I was supposed to get all better:

I didn't.

Just like when I took the antifungal medications, when I was supposed to get all better—I didn't.

Just like when we dropped thousands of dollars on acupuncture with one of the world's most famous acupuncturists—which most definitely should have gotten me all better—it didn't.

When I took the antiparisitic medications that were handed to me by an actual doctor, with a golden halo around them and the angels singing—when I was supposed to get all better and save all the women—I didn't.

No matter how high I jumped, there was always a ceiling. And the harder I threw myself against it, the more I got hurt.

I had told literally everyone that we had figured things out and I was on my way up and out of illness—but even as I was trumpeting it from the highest hills, I could feel a dark tremor down in the chambers of my inner knowing. Not-getting-better just didn't make logical sense. I had everything a sick person could want—a team, a diagnosis, and incredible faith. But despite it all—despite receiving acupuncture three times a week, despite the diet, despite being bolstered by hope, despite being held in the bosom of community, despite the birth of my inner artist—it did not matter how much I wanted to wake up from the bad dream. It was as if the Cheshire Cat had appeared yet again, rolling his smiling head, saying, *Not just yet, dearie*—before sending me off to the Queen's courtyard.

I wanted to be on the royal road to health.
I truly thought that's what was happening.
Everything I had learned told me that's what should be happening.

And as I sit here now, I don't know whether to laugh or whether to cry.
Because that's not what happened at all.

This is what happened.

~

I did start an epic romance.
It was with a punk rock musician, a minor legend at the Utah. He was handsome and bad, and he had the words *HOPE* and *WILL* tattooed on his left and right wrists.

That sounded about right.

In fact, after the diagnosis, success started to magnetize to me like iron ore. Everyone could see this was the beginning of my quickening return home. When my tests were confirmed four times by the Centers for Disease Control, no one has ever been so elated to discover a warren of pathogens living inside of them. *Strongyloides stercoralis*. A worm. A name. A creature with defined edges, a digestive system, and hundreds of sharp teeth—a scan to finally hold against the backlight. No chance of an unnecessarily demeaning name, like "Perceived Irritable Worm Syndrome."

I began to make preparations.

My life had been derailed in 2003, and I was ready to pick up where I had left off, just a short seven years later.

I took my medications dutifully. I continued to see the acupuncturist dutifully. I prepared to make a Wolf Larsen record—dream of my dreams. I set up a sort of writer's war station—books and journals and flash cards piled high—researching and writing about everything there was to know re: WOMI nation.

In my mind, I was ascending. My positive thinking was unparalleled. I'm getting better and better, every day, I said to myself, pinning another aspirational image to the vision board.

But reality and my vision board were not a match. As the months went by, I was still racked with pain, still required a colonoscopy prep every day, and I still crashed into a long, dead sleep every time I attempted serious reading or writing. My bones and muscles still throbbed. Other than grocery shopping and acupuncture, I could still do only one serious activity a week—having a friend for tea, or playing a quiet set at a club, or going to the Utah—but certainly not all three. If I did try to push it and maybe play two shows, joy of my joys, the toll on my health was enormous. Instead of going into a recording studio, I had to recruit a generous friend to engineer the whole album in my tiny bedroom, in my pajamas, in microsessions.

It took me about six months to face the dismaying fact that my body was not catching up to the rest of my beautiful vision.

The Universe had gone silent.

I could accommodate this invisible monster, as I always had—but this wasn't supposed to be happening anymore. The infectious disease doctor didn't know what to make of it. My gastroenterologist didn't know what to make of it and gave me a new drug for IBS, which made me worse. When I told my healers I was worried, they rapped my knuckles. Did I wish to fail my spiritual warrior training? No, sir. Did I believe I could get well? Yes, ma'am. I tied on my Karate Kid headband, set up my yoga mat, and smiled during the exquisite torture of Pigeon Pose. When asked how I was doing, I smiled, glassy-eyed, and said, "Better and better!" I was a doll, a string and pulley attached to my back: *Better and better, Better and better, Better and better.*

I eventually wised up.

Splashing the cold water of reality on my face, I decided I needed to take matters back into my own hands. When it came to dashed dreams, this wasn't my first rodeo.

I got this, I thought, looking in the mirror. WOMI, heal thyself.

With the clock ticking, I set to work. With dignity and determination, I planned a series of thoughtful, well-designed interventions I could do on my own behalf. Heal the gut? I could heal the gut. Maybe I had not tried hard enough the first time. So I took the best science and protocols from my research, changed to the GAPS diet, swallowed the glutamine, made the bone broths, took the herbal antimicrobials, prayed a lot, and waited. No change. Detoxify? I could detoxify. I went to Korean saunas, took charcoal pills, and applied clay packs and castor oil packs to my tender belly in my little bedroom while I listened to Deepak Chopra assure me in his deep baritone that "A is for acceptance," and "Y is for yes to life."

No change.

Perhaps the power of positive thinking, then? I was a positive-thinking ninja. I found several therapists who would help me search for the emotional origins of illness, working with the idea that your issues are in your tissues. The thinking there is that if you can uncover and work with any negative thought patterns, traumas, or unconscious self-sabotage, you can get out of your own way and let your body's self-healing mechanisms turn on. I'm pretty on board with this idea, and over the years I had done quite a lot of this work already (including The Work, by Byron Katie). I also found a regular therapist, as well as someone to help me with the Emotional Freedom Technique (EFT, or "tapping")—where you literally tap on your meridian points, work through different negative emotions and thought patterns, and counteract them with positive affirmations. For example, "Even though I hate that my vagina is on fire, I deeply love and accept myself." Some data indicates this really is a useful therapy for patients with chronic pain and chronic illness—a bit like self-hypnosis, supercharged with the power of the acupuncture points. Sign me up, I said.

Both of these practitioners immediately informed me that no bullshit would be tolerated. No whining. No boo-hoo I'm so sick. No casting the blame elsewhere. Full, 100 percent psychological responsibility. Accept these terms, or GTFO.

I accepted.

We began our excavation enthusiastically, and at first it was challenging, but rewarding. We looked at important things, like how my fears might be holding me back from going after what I wanted, or how my past was affecting me in the present. Then we started to get into stickier territory. *How have you created your own illness? How could this situation be benefiting you?* Difficult questions, but I accepted the challenge. *What you resist, persists,* they said.

The process was presented as a gladiator match between me and my inner demons, and I could either man up and slay them, or go home and stay sick.

And the therapists had lots of suggestions. Maybe I created a pelvic illness because I was afraid of men. Maybe I created my constipation because I couldn't let go of things. Maybe my body was attacking itself because I was attacking myself. Maybe I created my illness for attention. Maybe I created it to be loved more. Maybe I created it because I couldn't feel special without illness.

This was disturbing, to say the least. And it should be mentioned that this line of inquiry was not all that different from many of the self-help books I had read by authors like Caroline Myss, Louise Hay, Esther and Jerry Hicks, and Wayne Dyer. And it was not all that different from what many, if not most, of my alternative practitioners had suggested (if more subtly) along the way as well. However, each Rolfer, chiropractor, and homeopath had different suggestions for what my emotional problem might be—mother issues, father issues, core wounding, past lives, repressed memories, and so on. And indeed, it was problematic that they all had different intuitions as to what my emotional problem might be. And even more problematic that their suggestions always seemed to mirror their own issues. I ended up hearing quite a lot about my chiropractor's mother issues.

But I was willing to explore anything. Could I really do something like that? Create my own illness? I mean, what do I know. Maybe so. Anyway, I was a gladiator, and was there to do whatever it took. So I faced demon after demon, all the invisible scripts, repressed feelings, and a very real, repeated sexual trauma (albeit in a medical setting)—and for a while there, I was feeling like a right badass. Look what's down here! Look at all this junk! I liked shining a light on my shit. It immediately reduced my shit's grip on me, and I began to understand myself better. We looked at body image, and my parents, and my people pleasing, and my relationship to sex, and my fears, and my secrets. We looked at my personality traits and issues— from overachieving, to supersensitivity, to an elephant's memory for emotional pain. We looked at Dr. Damaskus. And we worked on letting go, letting go, letting go. It was all very healthy and very helpful.

But then, as we continued down this path for a very, very, very long time, I began to see that there was one vitally important catch to this inner mission:

There was no end.

There was only one way to "succeed" or graduate from this work, and it was to physically heal. If I didn't, then the only conclusion I was allowed to draw was that I must harbor more terrible thoughts that needed to be excavated and dispatched.

For example, if Shame was a big problem, which of course it was, we would tap through every Shame-riddled thought we could access—an exercise I found painful, but cathartic and useful. However. If I didn't miraculously heal, that meant either I secretly wanted to hold on to my shame—or that the problem was a different emotion, like Guilt. Following this logic, we would need to talk again about all the reasons I might have called my daymare down upon myself on purpose, for hidden reasons—as we tapped through every experience I have ever felt of Guilt. This was another painful archaeological exercise, if somewhat cathartic and useful. But, as my body remained unchanged, we would have to then move on to Anger. Then Rage. Then Sadness. Then Grief. Then Jealousy. Then Fear. And then around again. Rage again. Sadness again. Grief, Jealousy, and Fear—again. And then again. For months and months and months.

It was another caucus race—no beginning, no end.

If I still had pain and illness in my body, unfortunately the only conclusion to be drawn was that I still had a dark turn of mind. That's just how it works. Law of Attraction, and all that. We would have to keep digging, because if I wasn't healing, I must be lying, or repressing, or enjoying my infirmity.

So we hunted and hunted and hunted, and tapped and tapped and tapped. And to my ever-growing shame, I did not heal.

And slowly but very surely, as the months went by, this track of therapy began to have the opposite of the intended effect. I was starting to feel deeply, profoundly, irreversibly bad about myself. Slowly but very surely, I watched my inner, brave Katniss Everdeen turn around, lift her bow, and take aim directly at me.

This was the beginning of the end.

~

I wanted to keep at this emotional work like a good girl, like a good gladiator, but the months were flying by and I also needed to attend to more tangible measurements and interventions—which I was also failing at. I retested for the parasite, which was still there. I took course after course of the prescription antiparisitics, which, after a small bump in improvement, precipitated a steep decline in my health. Actually, whenever I took any medication, the boulder I was pushing up the mountain seemed to push back harder. I was starting to spiral downward, again, and when I looked into my affirmation-adorned mirror (*I am strong, I am healthy, I am Love*), I could see the desperation creeping into my eyes. I knew that feeling intimately, but I wouldn't accept it. I was supposed to be a warrioress, a positive thinker, and deserved an epic romance. I could not—would not—fail.

So I made a decision. After eight months of trying to allow the medication, holism, and the purification of inner demons to heal me—without success—I did what so many of us invisibles do. In order to keep up appearances, I wound up my trusted second self, sending her out periodically to smile, perform, and look pretty—but when I was out of sight, which was most of the time, I had gone completely and totally rogue.

~

In April of 2010, I checked into a fasting center, and proceeded to fast on only water for twenty-one days. I dropped from 130 pounds to 102 pounds (skeletal on my five-nine frame), when the fast was broken by a pillow-soaking nosebleed. I was so weak, I was unable to lift my head to stop the bleeding.

In May, I returned to San Francisco, continuing the fasting center's fat-free, salt-free, sugar-free, gluten-free vegan diet, insisting I was getting better. I spent weeks severely diminished and unable to leave my house without assistance, and was welcomed back to the stage by a Boston accent yelling across the room, "*Hey, Wolf Lahsen—eat a fuckin' sandwich!*"

In August, I worked with an integrative colleague of Dr. Andrew Weil, who commenced a full-scale war against my problem, including literal bucketfuls of supplements for my liver and my guts, medical food, niacin flushes, osteopathy, testing for heavy metals, stool screening, treatment for SIBO, treatment for leaky gut, treatment for candida, tests for food allergies, and treatments for any nutrient deficiencies. I knew these were all the good ideas for WOMIs, and I swallowed bucketful after bucketful for eight months.

That doctor insisted I was getting better—but I was sicker and weaker than ever, and the pain was starting to fan out across my back and down my left leg, its red flames climbing farther and farther up my spine.

Not knowing what else to do, I tried—again—to save my soul.

In October, I let the punk legend try to sexually heal me. (An extremely valiant effort, but no.)

In November, I tried to see if living wild and free could heal me, nearly drowning myself in whiskey, and blacking out in the middle of a sold-out performance.

In January, I worked with a clairvoyant.

In February, I did more EFT.

In March, I obtained my medical marijuana license and put it to use.

Absolutely none of these things did anything.

Feeling weaker and weaker by the day (but, I must say, quite knowledgeable about leaky gut syndrome, SIBO, heavy metals, the Emotional Freedom Technique, detoxification, and nutrient deficiencies), I left San Francisco for a final Hail Mary. I went to see a man in Los Angeles to undergo an illegal treatment known as intravenous ozone therapy. Intravenous ozone is a fringe treatment said to cure all that ails you, especially incurable infections—and we thought perhaps I had a particularly tenacious case of *Strongyloides*. The ozonator took me in, let me sleep on their futon, and treated me with IV ozone, rectal ozone, gua sha (a brutal treatment that involves scraping an ivory bone deep into your back to raise stagnant blood to the surface), and an all-colostrum (raw milk) diet. I only got a little bit better, but bent on finding the cure, not knowing what else to do, I moved to L.A. to continue this treatment. A little better seemed better than nothing.

In September, hooked to an ozone pump, drinking only raw milk, still feverishly trying to do more research from my pelvic sling (a homemade arrangement of pillows and bolsters set up to keep the pressure off the now white-hot nerve pain in the spine, bladder, ovaries, rectum, vagina, and left leg)—finally, severe panic, guilt, shame, and despair set in. At Thanksgiving, I desperately packaged the Wolf Larsen material my friend and I had recorded in my bedroom, and released the album before the walls closed in.

As I continued to fall slowly into the abyss, that record proceeded to go viral.

From an invisible cage, I gripped the bars and watched as my windup self took on a life of her own and moved on without me on YouTube.

At Christmas, my very worried family (the only ones who had any inkling something was terribly wrong) prevailed on me to stop the madness, get on a plane, and come home. I did not have the energy to protest. I needed help. When I got home, I slowly put on a green plaid floor-length nightgown, filled a cup with raw milk, and returned to my childhood bed. On New Year's Eve of 2012, I put my work in a drawer, drew the blankets around me, and stared out the window.

I knew what was coming.

~

Medical testing resumed with a newfound zeal and vigor—a thousand wires and probes searched out my every burning orifice.

Every hole was scoped, again. Every vein was tapped for an offering. Cameras were swallowed, radioactive eggs were eaten, and agonizing manual exams were forced on me again and again. Magnetic scans, specimens, doctors, fluorescent lights. *Ms. Ramey*, I heard a series of disembodied voices say. *Good news: everything looks perfectly normal.*

This time when they told me I was depressed and needed medications and psychiatric intervention, I sagged in my chair but did not argue. I wasn't depressed. I was destroyed.

All that fighting, researching, blissing, and writing—all left behind, along with my friends, my music, and my romance. Along the way, I had to break up with HOPE/WILL, the significance of which was not lost on me.

I agreed to psychiatric evaluation.

When I entered into another psychological workup, we walked through every shadowy hall of my psyche, again, and at the end, the therapist, now angry on my behalf, sermonized that I clearly had a medical condition, not a psychiatric condition. This patient, she said, is depressed because her pelvis, intestines, and spinal cord are on fire, not the other way around. She has not gotten the proper medical attention.

Hear, hear, I thought from inside the muumuu. But I was too tired to be righteous, and continued to stare out the window.

~

I suppose there must come a moment in every writer's life when she wonders to herself, Perhaps I should *not* publish a kicky memoir about my gyno-rectal disease.

I considered quitting the project, of course. Even at home, I was continuing to hammer away on my computer, sure that I was going to Really Figure It Out if given just one more day with my research, one more call to another expert, one more article on the

Internet about microbiota. I was sure I was going to get to the end of the investigative black hole any day now. I worked constantly, and though reams of pages flew from my fingers, none of it was quite right. I was still waist-deep in research, and up to my thoracic spine in rectal scopes and experimental treatments.

If you're wanting to reach through the page and put a stop to all of this, I don't blame you.

But it wasn't just obligation to the cause that kept me going. There was also the unmissable fact that I appeared to be more and more Right. This project I was working on was not just a creative, cathartic outlet (though it certainly was that)—doing this work threw light into a dark cavern where I desperately needed the gleam of knowledge. It had always been knowledge, not just positive platitudes, that gave me real, necessary hope. And as I lay in bed working, I watched as all of my crackerjack hypotheses and research were actually becoming really and truly mainstream. Even my father started sending me academic articles about the gut, autoimmune disease, and chronic fatigue. The Human Microbiome Project commenced at the NIH. Mold illness was in *The New York Times*. Fibromyalgia got its own drug, Lyrica, and suddenly people were taking fibromyalgia seriously. Michael Pollan himself wrote about the microbiome.

See? I thought as my hair started to turn white, and the mad scientist took hold. I frantically searched for a cohesive explanation. It was all connected—clearly—but the mechanisms were not clear. Just saying "It's the gut"—even with a solid description of what causes the loosening of the tight junctions between the microvilli, what perpetuates the low-grade intestinal inflammation, what happens when food leaks into the bloodstream, and the many consequences of disrupting the inner ecology—this did not a Darwin make. There were so many more fragments in the research, so many strange fragments—hormones, estrobolomes, the MTHFR gene, epigenetics, FODMAPS, biotoxins, mycotoxins—and somehow, they all belonged to one another, like a ten-thousand-piece puzzle dumped on the dining room table. Of a whole, but how would I ever put it together by myself? From the sling?

I tried anyway. One more journal article. One more book. One more video. One more training program. One more health coach. Each was a clue, and I tacked them to my research wall. The answer *had* to be around the corner.

But even as my research and hunches were validated externally, I continued to sink even deeper into my pelvic prison. I could not eat solid food, I could barely get to the bathroom, and once again it felt like having a case of the permanent flu. For days and nights from within my sling, I Sherlocked, and Scooby Dooed, and Miss Marpled for my life—turning over this stone, looking under that rock, interviewing this, that, and another specialist—wondering not a few times from underneath my mountain of research books, journals, and articles if medical school would have been a helpful first step.

But ultimately, after asking, asking, asking—writing, writing, writing—and sinking, sinking, sinking—I finally Harriet the Spyed myself into the ground. I had to stop, and had almost nothing cohesive to show for myself.

Which was not the legacy I had intended.

I had not produced the reassuring pamphlet I had wished for on day one.
I had not, even remotely, saved all the women.
I could see the writing on the wall, and it read:

Surrender, Dorothy.

And worst of all—worse than being a quitter—it looked like I was doomed to be just another WOMI, living at home with her mother, like so many of my mystery sisters, wandering from bed to bathroom to bed again in a green plaid muumuu and animal slippers. What little light I had been able to shed on my situation seemed to be going irreversibly out.

I was a failure and would be receiving an F in Nancy Drew's school for the modern female detective.

~

Around this time, a music video for Wolf Larsen was set to premiere on NPR. Good friends of mine had produced it in my absence back in San Francisco—a kind of offering to the infirm—but in a last-minute decision, the director flew to D.C. to get some frames with me in it. I protested. I cried. I felt too hideous, inside and out, to be caught on tape. I was too weak. But my friend was adamant: it was for my own good. If I could get to the doctor, I could get to the shoot. Put on some lipstick and get over here. After spending the day retching and folded on the bathroom floor, I pulled myself together, put on a pretty dress, picked up my dormant guitar, and tottered out the door in some high heels to go sit in front of a camera for an hour. We filmed, I hugged my friend for a very long time, I returned home, and I collapsed into a flannel heap that barely moved for several weeks.

When he sent me the final cut, my heart broke.
The director had done an extraordinary job.
There were string players in tuxedos, a stunning dancer, and magical special effects.
And there was me, looking back at me, through the screen.
As I lay in bed, wrapped in three blankets, pale as a ghost, I pressed my chapped lips together and cried.

Who was that girl with the red lipstick in the video?

I wanted to be that girl.
The girl in the video looked so pretty, so well.
That's all I wanted.
Not the sun or the moon or the stars.
Not a music video.
I just wanted to be me again.

It did not matter.

~

At this point, the candle snuffer that had been slowly descending over my head hovered dangerously close, and the light of hope started to sputter and hiss.

My mother came and watched me every night while I fell asleep, just in case.

She was as worried that I might die, as she was that I might take my own life.

It was horrible to see my own pain cause my mother so much pain.

Reader, it was horrible to still be alive at all.

11

Here, I think it may be useful to take a moment to pause and reflect. I want to leave Sarah where she is, and where she would lie suspended for several weeks. There are some important questions that one must ask, if one is interested in the truth—as I know you are, as I know I am. Of course, the usual things—what, why, how—*how*, surrounded by doctors and healers of all stripes, could something like this happen? Or, why did Sarah ever leave that magical acupuncturist, and her megavitamin friends? Or, how do we even move on from here?

These are all good questions, but here is a more interesting question:

Is this spectacular, spiraling, quest-induced flameout unusual?

Because the answer there is a categorical no.

The particulars of this common demise will be unique to the individual, but the pattern is not. When it comes to this kind of illness, getting a diagnosis is useful and such a relief when it first happens. She gets the long-wished-for name, a way to communicate to others, and a Wikipedia page of her very own. She is valid, she is real, and she has found the secret scroll to prove it. And not knowing she doesn't have the full story, she may very well trumpet her diagnosis from the highest hills: Celiac! Lyme! Epstein-Barr! *Strongyloides!* Look out world! I'm coming back! Finally, she is not a fibber, not an exaggerator, not a hypochondriac, and not a malingerer. She is a person, a good person, and the kind of person who is finally ready to be released, after years of wrongful imprisonment.

Preparations are made.

But then what happens when she applies the treatment and she does not get better? What happens when she is diagnosed with Lyme, she treats the Lyme, and she stays sick—also known as post-treatment Lyme disease syndrome, which is fairly common? What happens when she is diagnosed with celiac—but then she goes on a gluten-free diet, and she doesn't heal, which is also quite common? What happens when, in fact, she does all the right things and she gets worse? What happens when they put her on a steroid to quell the inflammation, but then all new hormonal symptoms start to appear—more food allergies pop up, deeper lethargy, more infections, more bowel problems, and more brain fog—and nobody, not nobody, knows why?

And what happens when the magic of acupuncture and yoga and supplements, if this isn't curing her, becomes completely unsustainable—moneywise, timewise, or otherwise?

Wanting to escape this crushing predicament is not a defect—it is the natural response. Of course we want out. Of course it is too difficult to bear. Of course we do everything we can to scale the walls, to get back to life as we knew it.

Because no one—no one—can keep up with the cost and the hours spent on full-time palliative care that isn't covered by insurance, that isn't solving the problem, and that could go on forever.

And if conventional medicine has no answers, or is making it worse, or is permanently demeaning and dismissive, it is human to try to find help wherever she can get it—no matter how extreme, no matter how woo. This is what sends people to ashrams, and cryogenic freezing tubes, and ayahuasca shamans in the Amazon rain forest. This is what drives people to set up in-home colonic machines, and become zealous about crazy diets, and too-passionate about kale.

That is how you get your rectum hooked up to an ozone machine at a stranger's house in the suburbs of Los Angeles. While these sorts of things are easy to pooh-pooh as a doctor, or a rational skeptic, or anyone on the outside—if you are the patient, the perspective is radically different. How do you say no to a cure? How do you resist the promise of feeling better, even if it sounds a little eccentric? (A lot eccentric.) This is doubly, triply, quadruply so if the illness has absolutely no protocol, no treatments, no markers, and no name. And it is quintuply so if your doctors are misprogrammed to see your symptoms as unimportant, irrelevant, or noisome. How do you not try to escape this nightmare?

It is a normal response to try as hard as you can.

And the problem is, this person's problem isn't normal. There is something about her problem that resists the usual narrative. Her smarts, her will, and her bravery have always served her well in life—but now it doesn't seem to matter how smart she is. Now it doesn't seem to matter how steely her will. Now it doesn't seem to matter how brave she is, or how hard she can fight.

Indeed, the harder she fights, the worse it gets.

Because here is the reality:

This wood is dark and deep, and if she doesn't have a map, a lamp, or a guide—no matter how hard she tries—she is going to stay lost.

~

Where we come back to our narrator, she is just so: lost.

Suspended in a black mire of depression, I lay in bed like a sack of potatoes and cried and breathed deeply and rolled into the fetal position, trying to calm my mind—a mind that raced between which wrong food I had eaten, which wrong emotion I was feeling, which wrong profession I was in, which parent was wrong, which wrong chemical I had let into my home—and on and on and on. There were no distractions from this horror. I had stopped working on my research, I had no bright ideas, and the doctors were out of options. I slept in the bathroom, took my showers sitting on the floor, and I cut my own hair.

I was disintegrating.

I really had no idea what I could possibly do to change this situation. I had done absolutely everything. This must be what I want, I conceded. *I accept I may have created my own illness,* I wrote on a sticky note and attached it to my mirror. *Take responsibility,* I wrote on another. *What you resist, persists.* I decided I just needed to accept that I was the attention-seeking malingerer those emotional healers had hinted at—the parasitic woundologist obsessed with being a victim, whom Caroline Myss had written about in *Why People Don't Heal and How They Can.* I didn't have a parasite—I was the parasite. Something was so perverted and so buried inside of me, no one could dig it up. I must not want them to, I reasoned. The hidden secondary gains were too, too great. There was no other explanation.

I am a monster, I thought.

~

The medication I was on was causing me to vomit out of just about every orifice, and as I retched into the toilet, nose running, eyes watering, self-hatred coursing through my veins, a thought passed through my mind, like an old reflex:

Sarah, you are really and truly In the Belly of the Yeast.

Looking into the bowl through a veil of my many dangling excretions, I let out a faint chuckle at my dreadful pun. It was the first chuckle to surface in a long time. Snorting a bit, I allowed myself just one more. I thought, *If this were a chapter, I'd call it* The House at Poo Corner.

Wiping my nose and my eyes of their snot and their tears, I smiled—a totally foreign feeling to my face. I pushed my wild hair out of my eyes, leaned back against the wall, and exhaled. It did feel good to make poop and vagina jokes again. I knew that girl. I pulled my phone down from the counter and sent my new ideas in a text to my longtime pun coconspirators, two fine friends named Colin and Ethan—who immediately replied, as if they had been waiting for the green light. *A Tale of Two Titties? Zen and the Art of Menstrual Cycle Maintenance. Speak, Mammary. The Cramps of Wrath. A Moveable Yeast. Infinite Rest.*

They asked how I was doing, and I told them it was a real *Snatch 22*.

I can't tell you how good it felt to laugh, even a little. Each bad joke, a hairline fracture in the ice that had frozen me solid. Just one small connection to my old friends, a gigantic bellows to my soul. I could feel the spell starting to break.

I got up to brush the acid from my teeth, and found a circle of sticky notes staring back at me.

Looking at the words I had written—condemning, terrible words—words that were not mine but that I had allowed in like a poison—I looked at these words, and from deep inside there came a roaring, rushing, unladylike sentiment of *FUCK YOU*, not to anyone in particular, but fuck you to the concept of relentlessly attacking myself in the name of healing, and fuck you to self-abuse in the name of soul-searching, and fuck you to damaging myself in the name of the enlightened path. I ripped those notes down, threw them into the toilet, and flushed them away with the last of my own vomit.

If I had an emotional problem, I realized it was that I had not said fuck you soon enough.

For the first time in a year and a half, I felt fantastic.

~

To be clear, I obviously believe in the mind-body connection, and the power of positive thinking. The mind has an enormous physiologic influence on the body, which we're going to talk about soon. Pity da fool who doesn't believe in the mind-body superhighway. It is well studied, it is well documented, and it is obvious.

But it is a *connection*. A two-way highway.
The mind is powerful, but not all-powerful.
This is at odds with much of the New Age, positive psychology, Law of Attraction, quantum healing schools of thought. The idea with those theories is that, wild as it may sound, you are actually in complete and total control of your physical health, that you have the power to puppeteer the function and dysfunction of your physiology, and you are not a passive victim.

It's an important, powerful idea, but it can become very lopsided.

If you are exploring your psyche to know yourself better, to understand your wounds and your weaknesses and your reactivity, if you're doing it to be less anxious, to be happier, to support your healing, to be more loving—more power to you. We should all be so brave.

And if you are exploring your psyche specifically in order to heal the body—this can absolutely bear fruit as well, I've seen it happen. People do quit their terrible jobs and resolve their IBS. People do go on walkabout in the Australian outback and go into remission.

But we must draw a line in the sand.

Anyone who is painting this as a linear, universal process, a 1:1, positive thought = positive body, negative thought = negative body, is leading you down the garden path.

One may be contributing to one's ill health with negative behaviors and thoughts—which is absolutely important to address—and one can always contribute to one's well-being and progress with gratitude, stress reduction, little joys, laughter, forgiveness, and love. Good gods—especially laughter, joy, and love! Which often, I notice, goes totally absent in the more New Age, "spiritual" circles, which are often weirdly somber and palpably self-righteous and self-congratulatory. But the concept of pasting positive thoughts over negative thoughts, or scrubbing out negative thoughts, or shooting at negative thoughts, or only ever having positive thoughts—all as a way of trying to push a button and get the gumball of a perfect body, perfect health, and a perfect life—well, where have we seen this idea before?

That's right. Everywhere.

Supplements, yoga, kale, chia seeds, Wellbutrin, Abilify—everything is sold as the Cure, the Miracle, the fishes, the loaves—and positive thinking is no exception. It is marketed like spiritual Paxil. Take two gratitude lists, and don't call me in the morning.

This is what I have come to call "Magical Pillthink," and it is our culture's Pavlovian predicament. We are all groomed, day in and day out, to believe that happiness—and now health and wellness—are available to you for the low, low price of a yoga retreat in Bali, or a positive-thinking seminar, or a prescription for Cymbalta. And especially when we apply Magical Pillthink to a person's psychology—and I cannot overstate how saturated the healing movement is with emotional Magical Pillthink—this can become very dangerous, and it can really do a number on your self-worth. Because the whole premise is: *you did this*. And that isn't an opinion; it's the Law. It is the truth, the way, and the word. And you are damned if you don't believe in this, act on it, and buy several courses on attraction and manifestation. Not getting better is a choice.

But this philosophy—which dominates the healing world—is totally divorced from reality.

The mind and the body are engaged in a *conversation*.
It is not unidirectional, mind —> body.
Without any question at all, mind <— body, as well.
I would go so far as to state the obvious: mind = body. Body = mind. One continually influences the other, and vice versa.

Inflammation, dysbiosis, infections, gluten, toxins—these deeply affect our brain and our emotional state, and cannot be forcefully overridden with affirmations and gratitude. By all means, we should all be grateful. We should all have a practice of loving kindness. I do. And this should be part of any healing program. But convincing the patient she has created her own illness all by herself for sinister, subconscious reasons may not only be really and truly incorrect—but, my goodness. Something here *is* rather sinister, and it's not the patient.

Hold on to this point. Because, as I say, it's not that this concept is entirely on the wrong track, and this will become more interesting shortly. I don't mean to rag on the energetic system, or the focus on getting better and better, or any of these things. They play a role—an important one—but it's just that, a role.

~

The larger point is:
That messy moment in the bathroom shifted something inside of me.

My body was saying something—and had been trying to say more and more things for nine years—and we just didn't understand it yet. This was too bad, but it didn't mean I was a big fat parasitic craven supermonster. Something was wrong, and attacking the problem with surgery and medication—or with a surgical removal of my darker emotions—was not the only answer. It had never been the only answer. I had been more than willing to offer myself up on that altar, again and again and again—and it just made things worse, every time. We were no longer attacking the problem—we were attacking *me*. That was the truth, and I was pretty much the only person who could or would stand up for that truth.

And so, despite the narratives that were coming in from doctors, the emotional freedom coaches, and my own inner mean girl—after my bathroom breakthrough, I just decided that no matter what it took, I needed to get back on my own side, Team Sarah. I needed to start thinking about what was *right* with me, not just what was wrong with me.

I could not—I still cannot—believe how hard this was to do.

And I have had to come back to this again and again when my health starts to go down the drain. Setting a boundary between what my deepest intuition is saying and what the Experts are saying, was, and is, essential. The Experts, to my great dismay, are not always right. And when it comes to this family of illnesses, I'd go so far as to say that they are almost always wrong. I don't want them to be wrong—and I don't have an antiauthoritarian, ideological problem with the Experts. I want them to be right! Help! But they aren't yet, and that's the way it is.

And so, what the patient knows to be true—this matters. What I know to be true matters. What anyone with chronic fatigue syndrome, multiple chemical sensitivity, fibromyalgia, Lyme, lupus, MS, ulcerative colitis, Crohn's—what they know, their experience, it matters, and the experts should be listening to them.

This is a very important flag for me, and for anyone to plant in the sand.
Not adversarially, but as an act of self-compassion.
And if she has been sick for a long time, this feeling may have run dry a long, long time ago.
But it is the most important thing.
Sick, tired, achy, itchy, despairing—she deserves to feel love, especially from herself.
She deserves to feel valid.
That is not asking too much.

And so.

This was the ground I reclaimed for myself, on which I could move forward, on my own terms.

I didn't have to understand—I *wanted* to understand.

I didn't have to prove myself by getting better—I just wanted to get better.

Not for a book, not for a boy, not for the WOMIs, but for me.

I figured this might take a long time, maybe forever, but for all my other maladies, I think immedicable hopemonger and incurable optimist should be added to the list. A part of me is tied to a rainbow hot-air balloon in the sky, and though it often drags me face-first through the hills, through rain and snow, and though my clothes and socks are full of leaves and twigs—God bless that hot-air balloon, and bless that unbreakable cord.

II

12

So I got back to my research, but this time: gently.

Not based on an outcome, and certainly not to Win.

There would be no more agonizing, and no more tearing out of hair.

The time had come to return again to sketching out my pet project, but this time around I went into my closet and pulled out actual sketch paper and a set of brush pens. Over the years I had learned so much—a staggering amount—but it was so much that now I needed to visually map it out on paper, to see if it had any kind of appreciable shape. In this art project I would also plan to include my own deeply unscientific perception of the problem, and for this I would need to consciously kill perfectionism. I would not, could not, be Carl Zimmer; I would not, could not, be Michael Pollan; and I would not, could not, be Malcolm Gladwell. I was different from them. I was not able to just be the observer, the clean, crystalline mind—because I was also the observed. Every time I looked into the microscope, I couldn't help it: there I was, looking back up.

And since I was the only one in charge of this operation, I decided I would not let my subjectivity be a mark against me. I would use my subjectivity. I would trust my subjectivity. And I would be comfortable with whatever came of it. In fact, I felt rather certain I was going to get Some of it Right and Some of it Wrong.

I felt a wave of relief.

Akin to what writer Danielle LaPorte calls "the euphoria of admitting your life sucks."

Tacking large rectangles of butcher paper to the wall for a blank canvas, I drew a giant, black question mark in the center, and I started to sketch the World of WOMI as I, Sarah Ramey, knew it.

~

The popular writers who line my secret library of health and wellness books frequently compare the human body to a car. For example, it matters what kind of gas you put in the tank to keep it running well. It matters that you drive it regularly. It matters that you keep it protected from the elements. It matters that it gets regular maintenance—DIY or otherwise. Certain problems are fatal. Transplants are sometimes possible, sometimes not.

All true for the body.

Personally, I don't like to think about humans as automobiles—but even if I did, this metaphor isn't quite right for WOMIs.

The sheer number of symptoms a WOMI drags around with her is so different from your normal illness, it is not like driving a sedan or a coupe—it's more like driving an open-bed eighteen-wheeler. Some trucks are relatively empty—maybe just a few Styrofoam cups rolling around in the back. But some trucks are filled with horses, or manure, or chickens, or straw bales, or lawn mowers, or onions, or broomsticks/rakes/ploughs/hoes—all manner of things, piled high and tied down with not enough rope—magnificently careening down the highway, feathers flying, disaster only a matter of time.

I thought this WOMI/automotive analogy (if I had to make an automotive analogy) was more accurate, and I started sketching.
It felt a little silly, but really, so does being a WOMI.
And anyway, nothing lifts the spirits like drawing chickens, lawn mowers, and manure.

~

Next, it was time to illustrate what I had come to understand as the WOMI Continuum. This was the center of my own personal research. At the core of my understanding was the idea that being mysteriously ill is not a singular disease, but a progressive condition, and characterized by the aggregate. It then follows that there is an evolution of WOMIdom, from zero to disaster.

No one else had verified this, but I knew it was true.

What follows is a map of the Continuum.

WOMI 1

This is the most common type of WOMI. She has mild symptoms—maybe one big thing, like asthma. This could be anyone—mom, baby, anyone. She has a few imbalances, eats too much processed food, does not have a wonderful balance of flora in her intestine. She has frequent constipation (or loose bowels), some skin issues, painful periods, and doesn't hit the ground running in the morning. She forgets her keys and her appointments often. She has to drink coffee to wake up in the morning, wilts in the afternoon, props herself up again with coffee, and then has to sedate herself in the evening with wine.

She is not Sick, but there are more than a few problems rattling around.

Note: this is what we have commonly but incorrectly come to think of as a normal human experience of life.

WOMI 2

Here is where the real WOMIs start to separate out from the masses and become aware of themselves as different. A WOMI 2 has a lot of nagging concerns—all of the symptoms from the WOMI 1 group, but now with terrible PMS, acne on her back and chest, low energy, low sex drive, a lot of yeast infections, and frequent constipation. She doesn't think of herself as Sick—but she is annoyed all the time with health concerns. Perhaps to the point of having to make an appointment to see any of the many doctors necessary to take care of her multitude of problems: the primary doctor, the gynecologist, the urologist, the gastroenterologist, and the endocrinologist. For each of these symptoms, there is a pill she can take (many of which create new, slightly less bad symptoms)—and if she doesn't take the pills, the symptoms come right back.

She, too, is not exactly sick, but she's got an awful lot piled in the back of that truck.

And if she doesn't tie it down with the pills, the whole lot goes sliding around, tipping over and spilling, making a mess every time she takes a turn too fast.

WOMI 3

A WOMI 3 is where things start to tip into illness. A WOMI 3 has all the symptoms of a WOMI 1 and a WOMI 2—but she is also noticing significant hair loss in the shower, throbbing wrists, and no desire to do anything physical. She may be in her twenties or thirties, and knows this is not normal. She has also become steadily allergic to a lot of foods. Not an anaphylactic reaction (no hospital visits), but she feels ill and very sensitive to things like eggs and blueberries and cucumbers and tomatoes and shrimp and especially (she hates to admit this) bread. She loves bread and does not enjoy this realization. She doesn't want to be one of those gluten-free zealots. But her tummy is bloated and she has started to wear shirts that blouse out around the waist to give her some room, regardless of her weight. She could be on the thin side, but sporting a babyless belly that looks well into the second trimester. If there is a bug going around the office, she gets it. If she has sex, she is going to get a UTI. If she takes antibiotics, she is going to get a yeast infection. On the weekends, the only thing she does is sleep. She has taken up with many alternative healing modalities, with inconsistent results. Her friends are concerned, not in small part because she talks continually about her health.

Now, not only is the flatbed filling up, but the automobile itself is starting to sputter. There are cracks in the windows, tears in the seats, no windshield wiper fluid, and the Check Engine light is on. She can hear animals starting to fuss in the trailer (where there were none before), but she can't bring herself to turn around and look.

WOMI 4

A WOMI 4 is a woman on the edge. She has fully admitted that she is sick, and she has tried everything—more things than she would like to admit. If she has the means, she has spent thousands, if not tens of thousands, of dollars on therapies and diets and supplements that have not worked. She is skeptical of everything, but cannot help herself from constantly trying something new. She just wants to be better. She wants to be cured. She would do anything. If it's not a magic pill from the doctor, she's willing for it to be magical Peruvian maca powder or a magical mini trampoline. She has started to work from home, and sits in an infrared sauna tent at her desk, stationed at her computer, with her arms and legs and head sticking out. She has a massive library of self-help and self-healing, secreted away. She has long since started to lead a double life, and rarely invites people over. She would be mortified if someone found out the full extent of her self-healing mania.

But she truly has no other options. She has been to the doctors, clinics, healers, and bodyworkers—and everyone says something different. Everyone preaches the Way. She has been driving around in circles with an overfull, extremely precarious, and malfunctioning truck, which no one will fix. Only one headlight works, the heater is broken, and the muffler is dragging loudly on the ground.

Passersby wonder why she's still going.
Some even offer to call roadside assistance.

WOMI 5

With a WOMI 5, the wheels are completely off the wagon. She's parked in the yard, decomposing. She is generally housebound, often bedbound, definitely out of work, and deeply demoralized. The truck still runs, it just doesn't go anywhere. There are no road maps, no protocols, and no space of understanding. There's not even a grim prognosis she can organize her life around. Just a slew of invisible symptoms—autonomic dysfunction (the automatic functions of the body, like blood pressure, heart rate, and digestion), loss of orthostatic pressure (the inability to stand up without getting dizzy or fainting), severe but unexplained bowel problems, severe chemical intolerance, severe insomnia, severe weakness, severe aching, severe fatigue—none of which means much to anyone else, but all of which have destroyed her life. She is in enormous pain, and it only gets worse every year. She can barely move. She has done every cleanse in the book, every healing diet, and she even owns her own colonic machine. If she had more energy, she could open an apothecary in her kitchen, selling off the many herbs, teas, and remedies she has acquired along the way.

But almost confoundingly, one thing is very clear about the WOMI 5:

Despite everything, she isn't dying.

That old saying "This too shall pass" no longer seems to apply. Indeed, a central, disturbing problem for a WOMI 5 is:
This actually may not pass.

And so, because she has no diagnosis, because no one can help her, and no one understands, she retreats for extremely long periods of time into total seclusion.

WOMI 5s are the disappeared.

~

If I have not made it clear by now: I am (often) a WOMI 5.

~

Let's drill down on that last point. I actually move back and forth from 4 to 5 and back to 4 again—even a few times up to a 3 (such as that blessed period when I lived in Maine, and even when I went to work for Obama when I was more of a 3+)—and this is an important concept. The WOMI Continuum should be understood as dynamic. One can proceed straight down the stages, from 1 to 5—but one can also move backward, often because of lifestyle and diet changes, which can get you from a 3 to a 1 or even to total remission of all symptoms. This process can move quickly or very slowly, even over the course of twenty years.

But for those of us who identify as extremely sick—as in a 4 or a 5—we tend to fall into a different category. Firstly, a major negative life event often precedes the unraveling. For us, and there are a lot of us, it begins suddenly—*bam*—something happens, and down we go straight to WOMI 4 or 5. One day we're fairly normal, the next we get a viral infection on vacation, and then weeks and months and years later we are somehow *still* sick, not just with viral symptoms, but with an entire eighteen-wheeler full to the brim.

However—and this is very important—the precipitating event does not have to be a viral infection, which is a mistake in the theory of the case that researchers have been making for decades. The drop-off can clearly be precipitated by *any* trauma—from a serious infection, to the loss of a spouse, to sexual abuse, to a skiing accident, to a Dr. Damaskus. If you spend any time at all in the chronic fatigue syndrome community, it is obvious that there is a much broader pool of triggers beyond just viral infections that can elicit the same illness. And it is also obvious that the worse the trauma is, the steeper the drop. In my own interviews with women, it was the fourth time someone told me that "it all started after that car accident . . ." that a cartoon lightbulb drew itself over my head. The specificity of hearing about a car accident in four separate case histories made me look back through my interviews, where I now saw that almost everyone in the 4/5 category started this way—with a major triggering event. It didn't matter if the event was emotional or not. The body had been traumatized.

And like the rest of the spectrum, this far-gone 4/5 subsection of WOMIs can also make interventions in their diet or self-care or alternative care in order to work their way backward through the stages—but it is generally a Sisyphean endeavor. It's very clear that once you are down in the pit, it is extremely hard to claw your way out without help. You may even somehow make it back to level 3, but if you don't maintain your extremely expensive, life-consuming health habits and treatments, the trapdoor opens again, and back you go to bedridden, housebound, and poorer many thousands of dollars.

~

So as I continued to generate this visual map for myself, I realized there was something I hadn't done yet—something I have not done here in this text, either, probably out of respect for the reader's delicate sensibilities. I'm always mentioning a lot of symptoms, a slew of symptoms, a morass of symptoms, a deluge of symptoms— but it's hard to know what that means, exactly. Because each symptom, on its own, is relatively minor—just as the doctors have said. Lots of people have night sweats—not to worry, darling. Everyone's a bit fatigued, aren't they?

But this is an illness of accretion. The distinguishing characteristic of a WOMI is that she can have an outrageous number of not-to-worry symptoms.

So here I'd like to present a fuller menu of symptoms associated with these illnesses, and this is leaving *out* the more specialized symptoms associated with the specific autoimmune diseases, or the specific infections like Lyme or Epstein-Barr, which have a much more defined (but no less miserable) set of problems. What we have listed here are just the mysterious pieces of lint our WOMI human-lint-roller commonly picks up along the way, for which medicine has no explanation.

Fasten your helmet.

~

At any given moment, a WOMI may be experiencing one, seven, twelve, or fifty-three of the following:

Flulike symptoms, permanently.
Polycystic ovaries.
Joint pain.
Painful periods.
Swollen glands.
Weight loss.
Weight gain.
Hyperthyroidism.
Hypothyroidism.
Fatigue.
Heart palpitations.
Night sweats.
Difficulty finding words.
Low blood pressure.
Poor sleep.
Short-term memory problems.
Decreased libido.
Racing thoughts.
Irregular periods.
Chest pain.
Coat-hanger pain.
Drug sensitivity.
Frequent sore throats.
Sinusitis.
Dry mouth and eyes.
Eczema.
Cold extremities.
Tingling, numbess, and/or burning.
Double vision.
Vertigo.
Vulvar vestibulitis.
Vaginitis.
Interstitial cystitis.
Yeast infections.
Day sweats.
Multiple chemical sensitivities.

Any of the one hundred-plus autoimmune diseases.
Dizziness.
Spinal pain (sacral, lumbar, thoracic, and/or cervical).
Vulvodynia.
Pelvic floor dysfunction.
Very oily skin.
Very dry skin.
Inability to digest fats.
Inability to digest proteins.
Rashes.
Urinary tract infections.
Kidney infections.
Paradoxical reactions.
Allergies (to any- and everything—from dust, to pollen, to cats, to perfume, to mold).
Hypersensitivity to loud noises.
Hypersensitivity to emotions.
Hypersensitivity to smells.
Hypersensitivity to light.
Diarrhea.
Constipation.
Alternating diarrhea and constipation.
Acne.
Severe anxiety.
Distention.
Irritable bowel syndrome.
Orthostatic intolerance.
Low stomach acid.
High stomach acid.
Postural orthostatic tachycardia syndrome (POTS).
Dysautonomia.
Bowel strictures.
Hemorrhoids.
Rectal fissures.
Rectal itching.
Abnormal vaginal discharge.
Migraines.
Trouble concentrating.
Gluten intolerance.

Cramping.
Dairy intolerance.
Sugar intolerance.
Gas.
Arthritis.
Fevers/chills.
Ehlers-Danlos syndrome.
Frequent ear infections.
Frequent eye infections.
Frequent bladder infections.
Every kind of food sensitivity (broccoli, strawberries, plums, pecans).
Insomnia.
Fibroids
Endometriosis.
Infertility.
Muscle weakness.
Mild depression.
Severe depression.
Cognition problems.
Suicidal thoughts.
Myalgias (aches).
Malaise after the slightest exertion.
Fatigue on waking in the morning.
Asthma.
Mast cell activation syndrome.
Frequent viral infections.
Bloating.
Heartburn.
Gastritis.
Rectal prolapse.

~

When I looked at this list, I couldn't help but think of every skeptic who had referred to these illnesses as the Yuppie Flu, hypochondria, laziness, Munchausen syndrome, or some kind of fad. And there are a lot of those skeptics. Many, if not most, people refer to the many treatments associated with this kind of illness (gluten-free food, probiotics, green juice, the paleo diet, etc.) as faddish, concluding that that's all there is to it. And while some of the commercial aspects of the phenomenon may be trends, the illnesses and the symptoms are not.

Jeggings = a fad.
UGG boots = a fad.
Beanie Babies = a fad.

Bedridden = not a fad.
Permanent flulike feelings = not a fad.
Crippling menstrual pain = not a fad.
Itchy rectums = obviously, obviously not a fad.

~

Once I started with this train of thought, I couldn't stop thinking about the problem of the ubiquitous skeptic. This topic is perhaps the sorest spot for all WOMIs—because it is everywhere, in every interaction, with every doctor, and even with friends and family, from real-life friends to Facebook friends—really anyone and everyone. The disbelief that pervades all conversations regarding the mystery illnesses is truly overwhelming.

But this is especially problematic for the WOMI 5.

Because imagine being completely disabled, experiencing sixty-two of the above symptoms—and also completely housebound, often bedridden—and having no one, often not even your own family, believe that you are really sick. It is devastating, and it is quite common.

And as I continued to think about these abundant naysayers, I couldn't help but recall what Dr. Nancy Klimas, director of the Institute for Neuro-Immune Medicine, who studies HIV, CFS, and Gulf War illness, said to *The New York Times* in 2009 regarding this common skepticism and diminishment associated with chronic fatigue syndrome. She was addressing a question from a reader who had asked her to stop comparing CFS to HIV, because it was offensive. And she replied:

> I hope you are not saying that CFS patients are not as ill as HIV patients. My HIV patients for the most part are hale and hearty thanks to three decades of intense and excellent research and billions of dollars invested. Many of my CFS patients, on the other hand, are terribly ill and unable to work or participate in the care of their families. I split my clinical time between the two illnesses, and I can tell you if I had to choose between the two illnesses I would rather have HIV. But CFS, which impacts a million people in the United States alone, has had a small fraction of the research dollars directed towards it.

Everyone should be aware of Dr. Klimas's sentiment. Virtually no one is.

And it echoes a statement made two decades earlier by Dr. Mark Loveless, head of the AIDS Clinic at Oregon Health Sciences University, who noted that his CFS patients scored lower on the Karnofsky performance scale than his HIV patients, even at the most severe progression of the disease. In his own words, he said that the severe chronic fatigue patient "feels effectively the same every day as an AIDS patient feels two weeks before death."

In fact, CFS ranks more poorly on quality-of-life review than renal failure, different cancers, multiple sclerosis, lung disease, diabetes, and heart failure.

This really matters.

Not because it is useful to rank terrible illnesses—it is not. It is indeed offensive when someone tries to make the point that AIDS is worse than cancer, or Lou Gehrig's disease is worse than AIDS. Because that doesn't matter. They are all very, very bad. No one would ever say to a friend with cancer, "Well, at least you don't have Lou

Gehrig's disease." Or, they should not say that and expect to remain friends.

But we absolutely *do* say that kind of thing to the chronic fatigue syndrome patient.

All the time.
Doctors do it. Neighbors do it. Friends do it. Therapists do it.

Ladies and gents:

I did it.

Before I got sick myself, *I* did this to a friend in college who had been recently diagnosed with CFS. Her parents had died in a plane crash, she had developed this familiar list of symptoms, she was really struggling, and I, twenty-year-old Sarah Ramey, was the one who suggested that my roommate see the school therapist instead of a physician. I believe I drove her to the counselor's office myself.

So, it is not just a common response, or the response of very, very bad people.

It is *the* response.
And it hasn't changed for decades.

And the main point Klimas and Loveless were making so emphatically, a point I emphatically agree with, is this:

It is the wrong response.

It is the wrong emotional algorithm.

And that wrong response has very real, very painful consequences for the sister, daughter, patient, or friend—not a completely dissimilar consequence than if we all woke up one day and decided to pretend that HIV/AIDS was not real.

And, of course:

That happened.

As most are aware, in the beginning, HIV/AIDS patients were treated atrociously.

They were treated as if they weren't there. And no one would study the disease. And no one would take care of people with the disease. And it was given a terrible, stigmatizing name. And it was nearly impossible to get federal funding to do the necessary research and development.

And that *only* changed because the gay community pulled together and fought back.

Re-fucking-lentlessly.

For decades.

In fact, they fought back so effectively that young Sarah Ramey spent her high school weekends dutifully sewing patches for the AIDS Quilt—but spent her college weekdays driving her roommate with chronic fatigue syndrome to see the college counselor.

And this situation has been historically true for many, many illnesses. Or to be more accurate, this situation has been historically true for many, many illnesses when those illnesses do not happen to affect straight, white males, and that is just the harsh truth.

And so, while I was lying there in my bed, curled in an unwashed ball, working these things through my very tired mind, I realized that the important takeaway from Klimas and Loveless wasn't just affirmation that my invisible disease was as bad as I thought it was—it was also an imaginary note, slipped into the pocket of my giant, plaid nightgown, signed by the many advocates of the many embattled diseases that have come before mine. And in clear, bold letters this note read:

Keep going.

And in tiny vanishing-ink letters on the back:

(Re-fucking-lentlessly!)

13

Looking at my wall, I felt darkly satisfied for having created an accurate, grotesque, doomy map. There we were! Connected. Graphed. Unvarnished.

This atlas had addressed for me one of the big challenges that always came up, which was how to avoid diminishing the complete devastation that is the life of a person with severe CFS or progressed autoimmune disease by equating them with a WOMI 1 or 2—at the same time as not ignoring or leaving out the women further up the chain. The Continuum made clear that calling the *entire* spectrum "chronic fatigue syndrome," as if it were all the same thing and had the same severity—which is very common—was the problem. A WOMI 2 is extremely lucky not to be a 5, and it's wrong to lump them together as having the same experience or illness. It's wrong for someone who heals her acne and cystic ovaries to tell someone who can't maintain orthostatic pressure or digest solid food just to drink more celery juice and buy a mini trampoline. But it's also incorrect to cut the black cord that ties them together.

Also, having fleshed things out to the best of my ability, I was starting to have a pretty good idea of how *both* traditional and alternative medicine were missing the mark.

Observe:

To the traditional doctor, WOMIs and our legion symptoms are basically an unfocused Magic Eye picture. Just a jumble of disconnected dots—minor complaints and faux diseases that have nothing to do with one another. The symptoms are so varied, so many, and so different from patient to patient, it all presents as a kind of white noise—pixelated, like a bad channel on the television.

They're just not willing to look at it long enough for the picture to snap into focus. Not willing to look with their eyes, but more importantly, not willing to look with their funding dollars.

And then in alternative medicine, the problem is almost the opposite. While these people do believe you, and treatments abound, what they tend to do is to *globalize* their personal, clinical experience. Whatever their modality, or their area of specialty, they think that's the whole thing. If they've decided Epstein-Barr is the problem, then everyone has Epstein-Barr. If they personally had Lyme, then everyone must have Lyme. If they are a therapist, *quelle surprise,* then all disease is rooted in the emotions.

Alternative practitioners are a bit like the three blind men and the elephant.

You know the story:

Three blind men walk up to an elephant, and, one by one, each is asked to describe the animal that stands before him. The first man carefully runs his hands over the trunk of the elephant—and in great, vivid detail, he describes a Trunk. Then the second man runs his hands over the tail of the elephant—and proceeds to give a long and robust description of a Tail. And finally the third man takes his time exploring the ear of the elephant—ultimately delivering a profound and lengthy report of a very large and important Ear. And each man thinks his description—the Trunk, the Tail, or the Very Large Ear—is the whole elephant. They are describing what they know, and what they know comes from their direct experience.

So, at least alternative medicine practitioners acknowledge there is an elephant at all.

This is a big step forward from being told you've made the whole thing up.

But the problem is, the patient might be a Tail, but the practitioner is treating her like a very large and important Ear.

They're in the right neighborhood, but they can't see the larger picture.

They believe that something is wrong, but each ferociously (and I mean *ferociously*) believes that his piece of the puzzle is the whole puzzle.

However, they do have one big thing they have in common with traditional doctors, and that thing is this:

If you don't agree with them, then you, my dear, are a damned fool.

~

Now hear me on this: just as I do not dismiss all doctors out of hand because they have treated me unkindly, I am also not suggesting that all of alternative medicine is a bunch of snake oil, hokum, and hogwash. Not at all. I am pretty sure alternative medicine saved my life, and those Louise Hay affirmations kept my hope machines going in the dark of night, like an iron lung.

My main issue, as I pondered, was that "alternative medicine" was not a singular discipline with a board of directors and a mission statement and a set of standards and protocols. Or, if you like: it wasn't Hogwarts, and there was no high committee of Gryffindors and Ravenclaws working from the same grimoire.

As I kept worldbuilding and looking at the bigger picture, what struck me most was this central point: I seemed to be one of a vanishingly small group of people who were trying to zoom the camera *out*, to see the bigger picture. Everyone I had found over the years who was looking at these WOMI problems seemed to want to zoom *in*—but I felt increasingly sure that this was a mistake. The more I studied, the more evidence there was that this wasn't a singular poison in the well. There was no one disease we should be trying to hunt down, quarantine, and obliterate for the greater good. There wasn't a single virus that had sneaked up the spinal cords of women everywhere. The problem was much more complex than that—a vast spectrum that had its roots in something systemic. You couldn't point a finger at some bad guy, because as soon as you did—you might find one pointing back at you, your own behavior, your diet, and so on.

Of course, that didn't stop anyone from pointing fingers—claiming This to be the cause, That to be the cure, and This Other Thing to be the Way and the Word.

The scientific and popular landscapes were incredibly noisy. All the keys of the piano were being played at the same time, and there was no score, no movements, and definitely no conductor. No one was answering what seemed to me to be the baseline questions you had to be able to answer: Why is this a new phenomenon? Why does it predominantly affect women? Why do some people get better with dietary and behavioral change and others do not? And how can such a vast spectrum of symptoms and diagnoses possibly all be connected?

Because at least to this one WOMI, laid out on her back, gazing up at the map—it was obvious that some explanation was connecting it all together, just as surely as Orion, his belt, and his shield.

What that explanation was, however, I had no idea.

I took a break and slept on it for another three months.

14

The first time I heard the term *functional medicine,* I thought it was some kind of mobility exercise with foam rollers and lacrosse balls and physical therapy. No thank you. Enough misprescribed vaginal physical therapy for a lifetime, thanks.

But there it was, *functional medicine*—popping up again and again.

I had to actively ignore it to keep it at bay.

I'd had my fill of theories, and to say that I was jaded at that point would be a gross understatement. When it came to people and their endless "suggestions" for things I should look into, I was beginning to feel less like gentle Sarah Ramey from the suburbs of Maryland, and more like grizzled old Peachy Anne Barnett, my great-aunt from the backwoods of Kentucky, famous for smoking a corncob pipe and shooting her sawed-off shotgun at unwanted solicitors on the front lawn.

So when I finally settled in to watch a talk about functional medicine on my computer, given by its most prominent spokesman, Dr. Mark Hyman, I was armed to the teeth with skepticism. I'd heard of him, seen his work here and there on *The Huffington Post*, and dismissed him as just another Dr. Oz celebrity physician—and so as he began his talk about twenty-first-century medicine, I almost clicked away. I had grown accustomed to twenty-first-century medicine referring to state-of-the-art technology, electronic medical records, and advancements in new surgical techniques. Bigger, better, meaner, quicker. Talks about the future of medicine tended to ignore chronic illness entirely, except to advertise pills to manage the symptoms.

But this doctor wasn't doing any of that.

He was talking about food and sleep and intestinal health and movement and social connection. He was talking about myalgias, autoimmune disease, chronic fatigue, and the nation's ever more irritable bowel. He was mapping out the whole, complex truth—and it was very, very inconvenient. I perked up.

The problem, he said, isn't diet *or* disruptive chemicals *or* guts *or* infections *or* hormones. The problem is all of these things. And any solution for the future would have to take it all into account, as systematically and compassionately as possible. Systematically, to keep things structured and efficient so both the patient and the doctor can avoid overspending, time wasted, and hopes dashed. And compassionately—he emphasized—because it isn't the patient's fault. Let me say that again: *it isn't the patient's fault.* What has become normalized in this country for diet and lifestyle, he said, is not normal. It is a trap, and everyone falls into it—including doctors, and their families. Following this, the doctor-patient relationship should not be a luxurious extra on the side—it is critical. Not just for the fuzzy-wuzzies and the group hugs—but because if we were ever to create a new normal and get the ship back on course, it would have to be the patients themselves who did the brunt of the work. The doctor needed to be there to be a guide and a tutor, but the ultimate point would be to empower the patient. *Docere,* noun: "to teach." And that *requires* a connection. The doctor's job isn't just to demolish disease, but to give the patients the real tools and confidence to make changes in their own lives. And perhaps more important, to give the patients the real tools and confidence to go back into their community and start fixing the problems where they had started—at the roots. Fixing cultural attitudes, fixing the food system, fixing insurance, fixing laws. If these illnesses were systemic—so was the solution.

By this point I was standing and clapping Hallelujah, brother from the back pews.

If so many years ago I had discovered my secret twin, my first WOMI—here, so far down along the path, it seemed I was finally coming screen-to-face with a long-wished-for hooded mentor. He proceeded to lay out almost everything I had been trying to piece together by myself for a decade.

~

Functional medicine, I learned, is about the root cause of chronic illness.

It is a special, standardized training that is starting to be offered around the country to supplement medical school for doctors and other health practitioners, focusing on the systems of the body. It isn't antisurgery, antitechnology, or antimedication, but the foundational teaching is that diet, lifestyle, and attitude are the cornerstones of health and that when it comes to chronic disease, you *must* start there. Specifically with a blood-sugar stabilizing, a microbiome-friendly diet, and a lifestyle that safeguards sleep, relaxation, exercise, and human connection as top priorities for a baseline of normal vitality. And the reasons for these recommendations are biochemical, not touchy-feely.

None of this is taught in medical school.

Dr. Hyman also explained—and this was what sold me—that the model he was proposing was not to be confused with what the public understands as "integrative medicine." He explained that *integrative medicine* has come to be a catchall term that can mean integrating almost anything alternative into the traditional medical model. In contrast, functional medicine isn't about giving the patient a goody bag of acupuncture, massage, vitamin D, and a quartz crystal as a complement to their Prozac and their statins. It is a very specific, standardized method for testing, treating, and stabilizing the four main systems that have been identified as the drivers of our modern, chronic illnesses.

These four areas of focus are:

The Gut.
The Liver.
The Immune System.
The Endocrine System.

(More clapping from the pews.)

But it was more than that:

The Gut, he explained, is extremely complicated. In modern times, because of a huge uptick in sugar consumption, chemical production, and antibiotic overuse, we are dealing with a very unhappy microbiome—and this situation is increasingly understood in functional medicine to be one of the direct and missing links to autoimmunity, and to the mystery illnesses as a whole.

The Liver, he went on, isn't doing very well in these modern times, either. Eighty thousand new chemicals have been introduced into the environment in the last century, placing an enormous and unprecedented burden on our detoxification processes. While not all chemicals are dangerous, and it is important not to become chemophobic, it is definitely true that a growing number of chemicals and pesticides are either known or suspected to have a negative effect on human health. And when the liver has too much work to do, it is unable to properly metabolize all the things floating around, such as hormones, biotoxins, certain chemicals, and any waste or debris. In some cases, these substances then recirculate in the bloodstream and may be flagged as antigens, stimulating the immune system, causing inflammation. In others, the recirculated toxins can get deposited in the tissues, which has also been associated with fibromyalgia, multiple chemical sensitivity, and food allergies. And in other patients, unmetabolized hormones and xenoestrogens can cause endocrine disruption.

The Immune System, he continued, and the many problems associated with immune dysregulation, is still not very well understood, as there are so many types of antigens, so many points of entry, and so much genetic and environmental variation from patient to patient. However, an overstimulated, dysregulated immune system has clearly been shown to be at the heart of autoimmunity and many of the WOMI problems. The focus for any patient dealing with these problems is thus to do everything in her power to reduce antigenic flow, and to cool the varying types of inflammation as naturally as possible via an anti-inflammatory diet and anti-inflammatory herbs. Many of the common steroidal anti-inflammatories used by a traditional doctor, particularly for autoimmunity, can cause major side effects—and most important, they do not address the source of the fire.

Finally, he added, the Endocrine System is extremely complicated as well. We tend to think of stress as a metaphor, but the stress response is biochemically quite real. Both stress and unstable blood sugar call on the adrenal glands to secrete cortisol to mobilize glucose from the cells when insulin has been tapped for too long. This constant call for cortisol disrupts the delicate conversation between the brain and the target glands. And as mentioned, some chemicals can disrupt the hormonal conversation in the body, as well. And when any of these conversations are thrown off for prolonged periods of time, you will start to see polycystic ovary syndrome, endometriosis, fibroids, hypothyroidism, painful periods, low sex drive, and infertility—aka the hormonal mysterious illnesses, aka HOMIs.

IBS, fibromyalgia, autoimmunity, HOMIs, chemical sensitivity.

I felt like I had uncovered the golden tablets.

And none of it was rocket science. But it was complicated, and I was relieved to hear someone confirm that it was complicated. The point was that the basic foundations of human health have been disrupted, and the effects of our new normal appear to be adding up to some very miserable, very related conditions.

There was not a magic pill in sight.

This was a system, designed to address the breadth of the problem.

And someone besides me was describing WOMIs—and not just the tail, or the flank, or the trunk. This was the whole elephant.

And he wasn't doing it with hand-drawn maps, tractor-trailers, lawn mowers, and conveyor belts—he was talking about a real system of medicine, with training and protocols and tests and research and data.

I was aquiver with that old feeling. The case was open again. It was what I had been looking for the whole time.

~

Because my hope was still in a fragile state, I immediately did a background check. I wanted to see who Dr. Mark Hyman really was, and I was thoroughly prepared for him to be a glorified massage therapist from San Diego. I was out of luck. Dr. Hyman was Bill Clinton's doctor, had been the doctor for the whole Clinton family, and sat on the board of the Center for Functional Medicine at the Cleveland Clinic—one of the most prestigious clinics in the world.

I went on to find that there was an entire army of doctors and practitioners who were associated with functional medicine, such as Dr. Sara Gottfried, who trained at MIT and then at Harvard Medical School, and Dr. Alessio Fasano (whose work on gluten intolerance I was already a fan of), who is the chairman of pediatric gastroenterology at Harvard Medical School and Massachusetts General.

Not exactly a bunch of slouches.

And as I looked back through my health library, I was surprised to find that several of my favorite thinkers in the health world mentioned in their books—almost offhandedly—that what they were practicing was a form of functional medicine. I hadn't really noticed, because except for Dr. Hyman, the concept of functional medicine as something new and different was barely a footnote in their books. But to *me*, this seemed like the absolute most important detail, because it indicated a *system*, not an individual's hypothesis. For years, all that had been available to me were the hundreds of individual hypotheses that I was tenuously, timidly stitching together, trying to make sense of things.

And who was I to say? I had no desire to add to the noise with yet another idiosyncratic theory of the case.

Because when it comes to the WOMI masses, I would argue that what we need more than anything is a *system* of care—the right set of algorithms—not just a wonderful joke-telling artist and empath, and not just a few centers studying CFS in Utah and California.

We need a grimoire, with a high council of Ravenclaws and Gryffindors.

We need a grand, unifying theory.

Or, at least a plausible attempt at a unifying theory—something notably absent in both conventional and alternative medicine.

That's exactly what this was.

And it stated:

Our endocrine system, our detoxification system, our immune system, and our gut are four sleeping giants that we are not meant to wake up—but they clearly *are* awake, and they have a very complex interplay with one another. And this cacophony requires the attending physician to understand it as a whole, not just piece by piece. The system of medicine that Dr. Hyman was advocating provided a general medical map of an incredibly complex problem—which he *acknowledged* was a complex problem, with no one-size-fits-all solution.

Was it a perfect system, or one free from the usual criticisms coming from conventional medicine? Of course not. Is there any system of care outside the bounds of conventional medicine that is free from its usual criticisms? No there is not. But Mark Hyman and I definitely seemed to have gotten our soapboxes from the same factory, and to me, this was thrilling.

However, the very best bit of all, Dr. Hyman and the rest of these experts were not me. They weren't some random CFS patient with an outrageous case of vulvodynia, lying on her bed, graying and exhausted, trying to solve the entire WOMI Problem by herself with posterboard and a Sharpie.

These were scientists, researchers, and physicians.

Finally, the cavalry had arrived.

~

I found myself the closest thing I could to a functional medicine doctor, posthaste.

And actually, it was the great alternative medicine pooh-pooher himself, my father, who found her first. He said, gently, that he did not know much about what she did, but she was widely considered the best gastroenterologist for women in the Washington area. And that he knew she agreed with me about my theories regarding intestinal permeability, the health of the gut, and the power of nutrition to heal.

And wouldn't you know it: when I got to her office, I found that this doctor was not fringe at all. She was trained at Yale and Columbia, and lectured at Georgetown. She was tall, beautiful, brilliant, and as well pedigreed as they come. Her knowledge of gluten-related disorders and the microbiome wasn't instead of her good standing as a Western physician, it was in addition.

But by far her most distinguishing feature was that she sat and listened to my case history for *two hours*. When I worried I was rambling, she asked me to say more. Say more? I broke down in tears—not out of sadness, but because for the first time in the long history of my medical care, a medical doctor had actually made the time to truly listen.

She wasn't a true functional medicine doctor (she was not certified), but she was an integrative doctor specifically practicing many of the principles of gut healing, gentle detoxification, dietary intervention, and lifestyle oversight—and this was good enough for me. She promised to work with me, and warned it might be a long road. She said it sounded like a difficult situation that had gone treated improperly for so long that it could be difficult to wave a magic wand. I wanted to lunge across the desk and throw my arms around her neck and thank her, thank her, thank her. And all she had done was acknowledge that what I was telling her was real, walk me through her thinking process of what to do next, and map out what we would do if that didn't work. In essence, she had done the job of providing medical care, with equal emphasis on the words medical and care.

~

Working together, Dr. Wonderful slowly weaned me from my miserable all-raw-milk diet (something I had begun in desperation in L.A. because my digestion was so bad, and I had not been able to go back to solid food) onto a very soft paleo diet, consisting of slow-cooked meats, vegetables, and bone broth. Next we worked out a plan for me to somehow, some way begin exercising again. Even for five minutes. Then six. Then seven. We then made sure I was sleeping and practicing good sleep habits. And she also ran the necessary motility tests, MRIs, and GI tests, such as anal menometry and the always-pleasant defecography scans—all of which showed mild abnormality, but nothing that required surgery. We talked about different supplements I had taken in the past that seemed to help—mainly ones to calm inflammation, to help the liver detoxify, and probiotics—and she had me restart a few of those. She met with me regularly, and kept encouraging me to stay strong, to keep pushing gently at the boundaries of what I thought I could and could not do, and to stay hopeful. She wasn't paying lip service to diet and behavior—she was making sure I did it, just as one would prescribe and require physical therapy. It wasn't optional.

And like the little engine that could, I started to come back again. In my phase of rogue, X-Treme cure seeking, I had all but torpedoed everything that had helped me in the first place, like yoga and a nutrient-dense, grain- and sugar-free diet. Because diet, movement, and sleep weren't saving me completely, I had become cynical and left them behind. And I had fallen apart.

But upon slowly, slowly reintroducing these principles, within a few months I was able to attend a friend's wedding—an incredible feat, having missed so many. I was able to play a single Wolf Larsen show—a belated CD release party in a large, beautiful music hall. I collapsed after each effort for weeks, but I was still thankful to be able to have done it at all.

Virtually everything I was doing was me, not Dr. Wonderful, and they were things I already knew—but she was *guiding* me, encouraging me, and keeping me on track, and adjusting as we went. This relationship was extremely important. She was the first and only doctor not to kick the can down the road, or tell me it was all in my head, or push me harder than I could tolerate, or overload me with a truckload of supplements and protocols all at once. She was the first and only doctor to talk to me extensively about the complexity of chronic illness, the problems of the medical system, and the reality of the nightmare no one else in a white coat with a gold-leaf degree would acknowledge for a decade.

~

I do want you to just take that last word in.

A *decade*.

It took a decade to find a single, serious physician who would treat me and my condition with both compassion and knowledge.

And reader, I am one of the lucky ones.

~

Now, at the same time, Dr. Wonderful and I both agreed that my case was much more complicated than that of the average WOMI she saw in her office. The severity of the pelvic pain and the absence of peristaltic signals in my colon were highly unusual, and she admitted that I would need more than just the basics of self-care and the right diet to truly get better. She didn't know what was causing the excruciating pain, and didn't know how we could address it besides the many ways that had been tried (and had failed) already.

Dr. W. didn't know what was wrong, but she theorized that until the pain issue was sorted, I might not be able to make a full recovery. But crucially, she said she would stick with me, help me maintain at least a baseline of health, and help me keep brainstorming ideas.

And what simple, potent medicine that was.

~

We worked this way for months and months—and I made my way back up the Continuum to the point of being semifunctional, perhaps back to being a WOMI 4 or 4+—that is, back to being able to get my own groceries, join a women's group, and even able to play a show in public every now and then. And this was wonderful—incredible, really—given how long I'd been trapped indoors, mummified.

But then.
Then, then, then.
Then, there came the plateau.
My old, and very unwelcome friend, the Plateau.

And living at home with my mom, only able to leave the house once every week or so to say hello to the grocery clerk, but still saddled with so many symptoms—that is, released from my sarcophagus but still stooped and dragging bandages everywhere I went—was not where I wanted to plateau.

So on my own time, I continued to devour the best functional medicine books I could find to see if I could uncover any new ideas on my own. Many of these books were helpful, but they were geared toward different corners of chronic illness than mine. They contained good plans for diabetes, hormonal balance, weight loss, and even autoimmunity. But no one was writing books about my end of the spectrum, the Disappeared. There wasn't very much about severe pain, or severe exhaustion. If pain or severe exhaustion was mentioned, it was more of a cautionary note: don't let this happen to you. I was used to this, but disappointed. The cavalry had arrived, but I was still in the dungeon, looking up with sad eyes as they trampled by overhead. My personal glass ceiling was still there.

There had to be a missing key.

I knew it. The benevolent GI knew it. My family knew it.

Why could I not heal? Why did I actually get worse every time I threw myself headlong into anything—a project, a healing regimen, a boyfriend? Other people seemed to get better when they did things like that—when they did what they loved, and applied healing protocols, and found exciting, tattooed lovers. Even with the new model of medicine I had been praying for, my body remained in partial collapse, and no one could tell me why.

Don't give in, I told myself. *There is an answer. There has to be an answer. You are very close.*

And I was.

15

The time has come to introduce the concept of the Orchid Child.

The Orchid Child theory, derived from the Swedish idiom *orkide-barn*, is the theory in psychology that between 15 and 20 percent of any animal population—from humans to dogs to mosquitoes—is genetically more sensitive to the environment around them than the rest of their species. They feel more deeply, and are more affected by sensory stimuli. The same is true of the plant kingdom—about 80 percent of plants can thrive with the basics of sunlight, earth, and water—but 20 percent are significantly more sensitive to their environment, and need both protection and concentrated attention in order to thrive. Here is Susan Cain, author of *Quiet*, on the subject:

> Many Introverts are also "highly sensitive," which sounds poetic, but is actually a technical term in psychology. If you are a sensitive sort, then you're more apt than the average person to feel pleasantly overwhelmed by Beethoven's "Moonlight Sonata" or a well-turned phrase or an act of extraordinary kindness. You may be quicker than others to feel sickened by violence and ugliness, and you likely have a very strong conscience.

In one sense, it is a weakness—a neediness, a vulnerability. In another sense, if we take plants for an example, these sensitive plants, the 20 percent that need the extra care and attention, are often the ones that go on to produce the most exquisite blooms. For example, orchids. The theory is that the same is true for humans, and it is especially evident in children. There are "dandelion children," who are on one end of the spectrum, much hardier and able to thrive in most situations. They show strong leadership and direction, but they may lack some empathy, or a sensitivity to the world and emotions around them. And then there are "orchid children," who wither on the vine if they are not protected, or don't learn to protect themselves—but if they are well watered and well tended, they grow up to be our productive artists, philosophers, aesthetes, healers, counselors, dancers, writers, and musicians. In the middle, you have the majority of people, who are a little bit of both.

I am a textbook orchid child.

Super-sensitive, I am the kind of person who can feel (and is affected by) even the subtlest emotion emitting from every person in the room, like a synesthete can see different colors for every letter of the alphabet. But I am also the kind of sensitive who wilted on the vine, and only started watering myself when I was forced to by illness. As a child, I ate the same standard American diet as everyone else, I pushed myself to the edge repeatedly in school, I was not very emotionally expressed, and I had no idea I might be an artist. To be clear, none of this was presenting as a major pathology—I was just a hard worker, always pushing myself to be the best, best, best, and I wasn't very communicative about how I was feeling. I was "a very nice girl." It was only when I was benched by my illness that these needs and talents and emotions and expressions started to emerge. And even then, I never stopped pushing. I was profoundly sick, and instead of checking out, I took on a towering research project.

But in the course of my studies, I came to befriend and work with a woman named Ane Axford—a former WOMI 4—who was now pretty healthy, a new mother, and working as therapist and resource for HSPs, or highly sensitive people, which is another name for orchid children.

And around the time of my functional medicine discovery and readings, I discovered a long essay Ane had written for her clients about the Minotaur's labyrinth of medical problems they might be facing as highly sensitive people. It was just like my map, and Dr. Hyman's map. It was about dysbiosis, adrenals, inflammation, diet, sensitivity, stress, toxins, nutrients. The great Venn diagram in the sky. Someone else could see it. I cried when I read it (classic HSP response).

She and I went on to have some very interesting discussions about neuroendocrinology. WOMIs, we had both noticed, were almost always—and I mean almost *always*—HSPs. I have never met a WOMI who didn't meet the full HSP emotional profile—extremely responsive to stimuli, easily startled, spongelike, empathic, and equipped with an incredible depth of feeling (good feelings and bad feelings alike). Ane and I had both always wondered if there was a neurologic and/or hormonal aspect to either of our mysterious illnesses.

Interestingly, even in the functional medicine world, hormones were at this time placed the lowest by far on the totem pole of significance. The liver and the gut were seen as primary, which can also be seen in the ways these things have been introduced to the popular culture—first the detoxification wave (juicing, colonics, saunas, supplements), then the age of the microbiome (which we've been in for a few years—probiotics, fecal transplants, bone broth, fermented foods), and finally a hormonal awareness wave, which is percolating right now.

But this broad awareness was not there in the early days of my studies—and so throughout my health travels, my blackout-painful periods, irregular cycles, and cystic ovaries were the least of everyone's concern, including mine. I barely even brought them up with doctors, because I knew mentioning them would give them a reason to press the eject button and send me to a gynecologist. Then the gynecologist would tell me that lots of women have painful periods, irregular cycles, and cystic ovaries—not to worry—and I should start birth-control pills. (Which I did, which always caused just as many problems as they solved.)

No one was interested in how my unhappy hormones played into the bigger picture.

Girl stuff. Normal stuff.

Over time, I had stopped worrying about it too.

Just another hornet in the nest, I thought.

I also thought that if anyone was going to know whether or not her endocrine system was involved, it would be me. After all, I am the daughter of a practicing endocrinologist, and the granddaughter of a very famous, very female, very feminist endocrinologist. We would have known if there was an endocrine problem. Right?

~

In April of 2013, I sank to the floor of my kitchen, holding a new sheet of lab results in my trembling hands. I could not believe what I was looking at. I went to my bed, set up the pelvic sling, and immediately wrote a letter to Ane:

~

Dear Ane,

This is going to come out in a long tumble, but you're the only one who can hear it, Obi Ane Kenobi.

I noted that writing this letter felt like a conspiratorial meeting between Scooby, Shaggy, Thelma, and the rest of the gang in the back of the Scoobymobile, doing our darndest to solve the secret of the old clock.

About a month ago, I wrote, *I told you about a functional medicine doctor, Dr. Tests.*

After months of work with the beautiful Dr. Wonderful in Washington, I had made a decision to move to Tucson, Arizona. I would keep up with her program, but also transition to a warm, dry climate, where I always felt better—and where I could do my pelvis a favor by wearing dresses year-round. I was very anxious to try to establish myself again as an independent adult—I was thirty-two, after all—and because of the Wonderful work the doctor and I had done together, I was at least able to take care of myself again. For me, this often feels like all I can really ask for—feats of strength, like cooking my own food and doing my own laundry. So with my mother's help, I moved. And I did do well in the dry climate, and spent several months making some new friends and trying to set up a new, semi-able life.

But of course, I did not wish to give up completely on finding someone who could help me get to the next level of health—inextinguishable hope, and all that.

Dr. Tests was a new functional medicine doctor I had found who would see me remotely, and he also saw the Venn diagram. But his practice stood apart from most others I had found so far because he based his work rigorously around the *testing* of female hormones, stool samples, liver function, underlying infections, and especially cortisol levels—with major emphasis on using *good* tests. Testing and measuring have always been the Achilles' heel of alternative medicine, because for so long reliable tests have been woefully hard to come by. (See: serious funding; see: serious research.) If you see a functional medicine doctor now, in 2020, they will use better tests—but back when this was unfolding for me in 2012, proceeding without lab work was common, with the main focus being on patient feedback instead. This is what I had done with Dr. Wonderful—and even though that was better than not doing anything at all, flying blind is not nearly as good as proceeding with some cold, hard data.

So I had found Dr. Tests.

And Dr. Tests was different from the rest—because of the tests, yes—but mostly because of one specific test. In Dr. Test's practice and training program for functional medicine practitioners, he explained that there is one test that matters a little bit more than all the rest.

You must, he explained, test the HPA axis.
Or, the hypothalamic-pituitary-adrenal axis.

Adrenals? I thought when I first saw this. I had read about them, and knew the basics. The adrenal glands are a pair of small glands that sit on top of the kidneys. They are part of the endocrine system, and they are the glands that secrete glucocorticoids (predominantly cortisol) and adrenaline in your body. Your hypothalamus and pituitary are the glands that tell the adrenals when to do so, and how much. And the adrenal glands' most famous function is the fight-or-flight response. When faced with danger, the body immediately begins to secrete both adrenaline and cortisol, a series of chemical reactions that help you fight, freeze, or take flight. The adrenals, the hypothalamus, and the pituitary function as your stress mediators.

Sure, sure, I thought.
"Stress."
I already knew that.
Yoga. Pranayama. Meditation. Wind chimes. Got it.

So at first I thought this guy might have a touch of Very Large Ear Syndrome, focusing too much on only one part of the elephant. Oh *really*, Dr. Tests? I'd like to hear why the adrenals are so important? Ahead of, say, the gut?

He went on to explain that the HPA axis controls a rhythmic, hormonal conversation that is happening in the body all the time. The hypothalamus scans the body, decides if the adrenals need to secrete any hormones; if they do, it sends the message to the pituitary, which talks to the adrenals, and voilà: secretion. Cortisol. ACTH. Adrenaline.

In a normal state, cortisol and adrenaline are called on throughout the day to buffer and address any small stresses that come up. The system can also go into high gear, built to help you cope with occasional major stress or trauma, as well. And most people have usually heard the following explanation of stress: back in the day, our big stressors would have been the chance grizzly bear, an unexpected saber-toothed tiger, drought, famine, winter, and so on. Modern life has protected us from many of these more dramatic stressors of the wild, but of course we have replaced them with our own new stresses. Modern people experience two different types of traumas—big T and little t. Big T traumas include things like rape, domestic abuse, combat, the unexpected death of a spouse, acrimonious divorces, major infections, head injuries, and accidents. And then there are traumas with a little *t*. Losing a job, a bad breakup, and a move to a new city are some little *t* examples.

All of the above are called "external stressors." They all activate the HPA axis, and the production of the stress hormones, especially cortisol.

This comprises most of our normal understanding of "stress."

However, big *T* and little *t* stressors aren't the only triggers for cortisol production.

When you eat a high-glycemic meal, blood sugar goes up, insulin moves the glucose to the cells, blood sugar then drops—and the *drop* causes cortisol and other glucocorticoids to be secreted to bring blood sugar back up to baseline. The same is true for chronically high blood sugar, as in diabetes. When sugar does drop, it is cortisol that comes in to stabilize things. And in the West, we consume a famously high-glycemic, low-fiber diet—read: a lot of blood sugar spikes and drops throughout the day, calling on small amounts of cortisol, insulin, and leptin all day, every day. This is a very modern phenomenon.

And this same constant biochemical call for small amounts of cortisol will be triggered if you maintain *low* blood sugar all day, as in the woman who eats a few almonds for breakfast, salad for lunch, and salad for dinner, and keeps herself going all day with Diet Coke, Provigil, and coffee. Disordered eating, low blood sugar, smart drugs, and caffeine all register as stress, and all stimulate cortisol production.

Another trigger is sleep deprivation. Reducing sleep by even one hour—and certainly two, three, or four hours short of the recommended eight—primes the amygdala (the fear center) to be much more reactive the next day. Fear activates the HPA axis.

Another trigger is inflammation. Infections, food sensitivities (especially to gluten), inflammatory foods, toxins, mold, heavy metals, and inflammatory diseases—all inflammation is registered as stress in the body and all inflammation will rev the HPA axis.

Another trigger is pain. Unremitting pain is *extremely* stressful, and to this one I can attest.

All of these—unstable blood sugar, sleep deprivation, infections, inflammation, pain—are called "internal stressors." They activate the HPA axis without much conscious input.

Then finally, in the last category are the everyday stresses and issues that generally constitute the rest of our common, cultural understanding of stress. We know what these are: horrible bosses, traffic jams, social media, deadlines, debt, constant connection to technology, bringing work home, negative news, toxic relationships, body-image problems, and so on. We have a lot of this in our culture. And, of course, we all already know about this kind of stress and that we should be "less stressed." These kinds of everyday issues are especially problematic for those of us of the HSP persuasion—these problems are known to cause significantly more distress for us, just because of our wiring. We jangle easily, and it is such a jangly world.

And this common, culturally understood category of stress is counted as both internal and external. Much of it is happening outside of you, but some of the stress response is largely within one's control. It is called "perceived stress" because life is not actually in danger, and there is no real need to fight, or take flight. With work, these things can be dealt with personally. One can change one's environment to be less stressful, or change the quality of one's response. Serenity now, and so on.

But if we look at this list, we see something very important:

Horrible bosses and bad body image are not our only stressors. Having an infection is not a matter of perception, or serenity.

The HPA axis can be thought of as home to a small red emergency button. Negativity, your boss, deadlines, and social media can all certainly push that button—but problems with the diet, gut dysbiosis, sleep, infections, toxins, and food sensitivities can also be pressing that same red button, even more frequently, well below the threshold of consciousness.

It is not a very different concept from the constant antigen activation of the immune system. It's happening, but you're not aware that it's happening.

And this really matters.

While most of these factors are not new—sugar, gluten, stress, dysbiosis—what *is* new is the sheer volume at which they exist in modern society. All of the stressors listed above are a pretty good description of the new normal. Our encounters with these things are not chance—they're constant.

The average American consumes roughly sixty-six pounds of sugar annually—orders of magnitude more than the amount of sugar an average American consumed just a hundred years ago. Not only is that a lot more sugar—it is a lot more cortisol.

The average American gets two hours less sleep than the average American did a hundred years ago. That has many consequences, and one of them is a more reactive amygdala, and thus more cortisol.

Infections have always been around, but since we have succeeded so profoundly with treating acute infections—saving millions and millions and millions of lives—chronic use of antibiotics have also opened the doorway to chronic infections, resistant infections, and most importantly (in combination with a high-sugar diet): gut dysbiosis. This is a major, major new stressor—and most people have never even heard the word "dysbiosis."

But it doesn't end there. As mentioned before, the average American has been exposed to eighty thousand new chemicals in the environment over the last century, and the number continues to grow. While a little contact is okay, or even a moderate amount, an onslaught is not okay. And it's not just the big bad wolves like pesticides and BPAs; there are also toxins in our medications, our baby wipes, our makeup, our mattresses, and our new clothes. There are toxins everywhere. This creates a real burden on the body. Cortisol.

Food sensitivities, especially to gluten (to everyone's dismay), have become extremely widespread. More about this later on, but for now just understand this: when the IgA (immunoglobulin A) immune response is activated in response to gliadin proteins in the bloodstream, so is the stress response.

And, as we hear every day in our news feeds (omnipresent news feeds, mostly bad news, which also compounds the problem), we now live in a relentlessly go, go, go world, full of screens, and late nights, and folks who don't quite know how to turn off. Stress. Cortisol.

As a people, we tap that emergency button all day, every day, and we don't know it.

Thus the development of a problem with the red button is perhaps fairly predictable. The HPA axis is not an unbreakable machine, it is a delicate system in the body. While it is resilient, it isn't immortal. It can handle stress just fine—just not constant stress, from every direction, all the time. It makes sense that it might get confused. We're not supposed to have constant stress, from every direction, all the time.

And this confusion is thought, by Dr. Tests and others, to lead to a phenomenon known as dysregulated cortisol.

This is sometimes called "adrenal fatigue," but we aren't going to call it that. For one, just like its friends gluten and dysbiosis, that phrase is already extremely fraught in the medical community, and not taken seriously. It is also linguistically misleading, as the adrenals themselves are not fatigued or damaged—it's the HPA *conversation* that has broken down. Either way, you and I are going to leave "adrenal fatigue" behind for now. From here on out, we're going to go with the terms used by researchers—*cortisol dysregulation* and *HPA axis dysregulation*. But all of the above, of course, are the exact same thing.

HPA axis dysregulation is quite real. There are thousands of studies on this phenomenon.

While the exact mechanisms are not fully understood, we do have a sense of the basics. After a very long time of being activated—all day, every day—the brain's hippocampus appears to shrink, and because the hippocampus affects the HPA axis, this means that the HPA axis stops being able to produce cortisol in its healthy, predictable ski slope of a diurnal pattern. According to Dr. Tests, a healthy person is meant to wake up with between twenty and twenty-five units of cortisol flooded into their system, which is what gives you a boost in the morning to hit the ground running. This slowly tapers off throughout the morning, and throughout the day—with small bumps at both lunch and dinnertime, tapering off to nearly zero at bedtime, which is part of what makes you feel sleepy. Of cortisol's many functions in the body, the main one is that it is in charge of how your body makes and how your body uses energy.

Graphed, the daily pattern looks like an elegant ski slope, with some moguls at the end.

But when this cycle is disrupted, the body begins to produce the wrong amounts of cortisol at the wrong times. This dysregulation will get worse as time goes on if whatever is overstimulating the axis is not changed or removed—that is, if behavior is not modified or the stressor is not eliminated.

That is, over time the problem does not remain static, it evolves.

It is dynamic.

It has stages.

In Stage 1, the person begins to produce too much cortisol— instead of a smooth ski slope production of cortisol, there is a surge in the morning, followed by a slight crash in midmorning, and then again in the late afternoon. Symptoms associated with Stage 1 are mild: slight fatigue, skin problems, mild hormonal problems, and possibly more bowel complaints than the next guy. Nothing serious.

In Stage 2, cortisol starts to be sky-high in the morning, but the subsequent crashes throughout the day are much steeper and require a lot more propping up with sugar and caffeine. At this point, cortisol also starts to go *up* in the evenings, before bedtime—producing a kind of second wind, and insomnia. This results in less sleep, and thus more cortisol dysregulation. Now she starts to see real problems—because excess cortisol, as with any hormonal imbalance, starts to disrupt the whole endocrine system. For example, cortisol dysregulation is known to lead directly to sex-hormone dysregulation. Dr. Sara Gottfried has written about this extensively. For just one example, cortisol takes precedence when it comes to engaging the receptors on any cell. So if there is a flood of cortisol, researchers have found that cortisol will hog the receptor sites in the body. This means other sex hormones can't engage at the receptor sites and therefore will continue to float around unused. If the brain gets the message that estrogen never got to the cell, then the body produces *more* estrogen, even though there is already plenty. Over time this can lead to estrogen dominance, which is highly correlated with PCOS, infertility, and endometriosis. This is just one example of an extremely long list of possible hormonal fallouts. Excess cortisol has been shown capable of affecting many other hormones—for example, testosterone, DHEA—and it can especially slow down the thyroid, and this is thought to be one of the main contributors to subclinical hypothyroid problems.

This is a lot, but this is not all.

Dr. Tests explained that when cortisol goes up, immunity is suppressed. So when cortisol dysregulation is chronic, *immunity is chronically suppressed.*

If I could gracefully write in all caps here, I would.

When the stress response is activated, the body favors systems that are essential for survival—it sends blood to the large muscles for flight, dilates the pupils, and increases heart rate. It draws blood and energy away from less essential parts of the body—for example, the immune system and the digestive system. If faced with a lion, your body is appropriately less concerned in the moment with digestion, or warding off the common cold. But if there isn't actually a lion—if you are just in this very common, very modern state of being stressed, sugar-addicted, caffeine-addled, wired, and tired, and have measurably high cortisol, you can be sure your immunity is likely not in a state of excellence, and you won't have nearly as many troops defending the gates. So now—not only are you feeling stressed, tired, and wired, with trouble sleeping, as well as worrisome hormonal and metabolic problems (like night sweats, hot flashes, cold feet)(at age twenty-six), but you *also* seem to be picking up every flu, every cold, and every sore throat. If someone is going to pick up a nasty virus on vacation, it is pretty reliably going to be you.

This brings us to Stage 3.

Stage 3, come to find, is almost always precipitated by a trauma.

For this person who has been muddling along at Stage 2, perhaps for a very long time—not really sick, but not really well either—when a car hits them head-on out of nowhere, or there is a huge, rancorous divorce, or a nasty virus hits, or they get bitten by an infected tick—this person's stress response is no longer able to react properly. This person switches suddenly from producing very high amounts of cortisol to extremely low amounts of cortisol. They fall precipitously off a cliff—but it is an invisible cliff, and an invisible fall. The exact mechanism that causes this switch is not totally understood, though it is known that the state of chronic stress damages or causes the hippocampus to shrink, which in layman's terms "screws the pooch" for further, appropriate cortisol production. Clinicians who understand this problem and regularly measure cortisol patterns in their patients all report the same phenomenon. Once the patient has been in Stage 2 for long enough, and a trauma is introduced, she is almost inevitably moved to this next level, which is a state of *low* cortisol. The adrenals and the hypothalamus and the pituitary still work just fine, but their ability to converse with one another properly has broken down. Now in the morning, the patient wakes up with well below the average units of cortisol—and accordingly hits the ground dragging. While excess cortisol has its problems, low cortisol is a much bigger issue. This low level stays low throughout the day, and she feels like complete hell all the time—she quite literally doesn't have enough of the hormone that is in charge of how her body makes and uses energy. Her sex hormones are all out of whack, she can't conceive, her thyroid is slowing down, and she has a very low sex drive. Because her digestion is so poor, her mitochondria are not getting the nutrients they need to produce cellular energy, causing even more fatigue. This is all creating more anxiety, more stress, a more depressed immune system, and she gets sick all the time.

Starting to ring any bells?

But most important of all:

When cortisol goes down, according to Dr. Tests, the hormone DHEA goes down—and the hormone DHEA is directly connected to how much secretory IgA, or mucosal immunity, is produced in the gut. Eighty percent of our immune system resides in the gut, and so when cortisol goes down, it brings intestinal mucosal immunity down with it. Thus: this person who is already saddled with so many health problems suddenly has a deficit of immune troops in her gut. Out of sight and out of mind, these troops have been defending and protecting her all her life from the inside out, stationed at the walls and ramparts of her intestinal lining. But when DHEA goes down, these soldiers are slowly put to sleep, one battalion at a time.

This is not good.
She needs those troops.
And so now, the real unraveling begins.

Now this Stage 3 person may be struggling with a serious infection like Lyme or Epstein-Barr, or a head injury from an accident, or the ongoing stress of a divorce—in addition to very low cortisol production and poor mitochondrial function, as well as all manner of hormonal problems (all of which, especially aggregated, is extremely stressful in and of itself)—*now* they also have a very unusual state of low mucosal immunity in the gut. And so now, when this person with suppressed secretory IgA takes antibiotics for her sore throat, *her own immunity is not there in full force to help her restore the proper flora in the gut.* She needs those ground troops to keep pathogens at bay, which gives the good bugs time to repopulate. Stated more clearly: the lady who does not have those ground troops in place is the lady who takes Cipro, and immediately develops thrush, a yeast infection, and diarrhea—whereas the gentleman next to her, who does not have a problem with cortisol or suppressed secretory IgA, can take a course of antibiotics and reboot his flora just fine.

These two people are mucosally very different.

And what this means is: the woman with suppressed gut immunity has become *the perfect host*.

And not in the Emily Post sense.

Now, when the gut doesn't reboot, and becomes colonized by too many of the bad guys, and not enough good guys, real and intractable dysbiosis commences, and the reactive inflammation in the gut starts to rage (a different branch of the immune system that is very much not suppressed)—all of which is exacerbated by poor diet, continuing stress, insomnia, and the enormous stress of being sick and addled. Here, in this swampy environment, in addition to everything else, this type of person can almost certainly say goodbye to healthy intestinal function, and hello to our least favorite syndrome, leaky gut syndrome.

And once that gate is open, the inflammatory, antigenic hellions are no longer confined to the gut and may roam freely throughout the body, like Orcs released from Mordor.

And by now, we know what that does.
The exact immune issue(s) she develops will likely depend on her genetic weak links.
Lupus, MS, food sensitivities, mast cell activation syndrome—these are all immune problems.

But as you can see, those intestinal gates don't just poof open on their own—and it doesn't happen to everyone who takes antibiotics. The upstream problem in the brain and the resulting hormonal problem set the stage, and make the entire thing much more difficult to heal.

Thus, in this type of patient, no matter how many heroic interventions she undertakes to battle this dysbiosis and inflammation—no matter how much she tries to suppress symptoms, detoxify, take probiotics, and affirm herself—trying to staunch the many, many, many, many, many symptoms that will follow—even if she tries to heal the gut lining—if nothing is being done about the HPA axis dysfunction, especially if she has progressed into Stage 3:

She cannot get better.

Glass ceiling, thy name is stress.

And because cortisol dysregulation is not considered real or important, it is thus a problem her regular doctors cannot or will not measure, and she herself cannot articulate. It is invisible. And it *is* related to her state of mind. But also to the state of her diet. And also to the uncontrollable bad things that happen in life. And also to the state of her sleep. And also to the state of her gut. And also to any infections she might have. Or head injuries. Or pain.

It is not her fault.
She is a product of her environment.

And unfortunately, a broken HPA axis is not "fixable." The hormonal pattern and the brain itself have to be retrained, and rehabilitated, and all the major stressors, internal and external, must be removed. An antidepressant, which is surely about to be prescribed (and to be clear, depression *is* a comorbidity here—but secondary to the problem, not the problem itself) can only help so much, if at all.
   A broken HPA axis has to do with the entirety of the patient's *life*—diet, dysbiosis behaviors, stress levels, infections, body burdens, and past traumas alike.
   A broken HPA axis has to do with the person, not just the disease.

It is inherently miracle pill–resistant.
It is inherently struggle-resistant.
And the more you leap, and push, strive, and fight, the deeper you sink.

Ding. Ding. Ding.

~

I remember when I first came across the description of the stages of cortisol dysregulation—first narrowing, then widening my eyes.

Stages?
A continuum?
A drop-off point that is impossible to come back from without help?
The near-universal prerequisite for a dysbiotic gut?
Hell on earth, and a torrent of inflammatory symptoms appearing all over the body?

Holy f___.

I remember looking at this graph, and then looking at my graph on the wall, and then looking at this graph, and then looking at my graph on the wall, and then howling at the very top of my lungs, like I had just solved the mystery of life itself.

~

To me, I wrote to Ane, *this is the missing link.*

This is the Lucy—the beginning of an explanation as to why hormonal issues, adrenal issues, immune issues, and gut issues have anything to do with each other. I knew they did, but only in an observational way, not in a scientific way.

It is the chronic state of compromised intestinal immunity which opens the gut up for any number of infections, general dysbiosis, and a leaky gut. This is directly related to cortisol.

Furthermore, as overall immunity goes down, the person is then open to ALL manner of infections (for example, Epstein-Barr, Lyme, Strongyloides)—that they are then unable to kick.

It is a porous state of being.

She is a sponge.

~

So, to recap:

The gut is often the biggest, most hulking problem, and the gateway to many of the worst of the symptoms—but according to Dr. Tests and a whole lot of others, it isn't the keystone.

For most people, the keystone is upstream.
The keystone is cortisol.
Or, more accurately, the keystone is stress.

Which is kind of bad news.

Because Stress is probably the concept that all of us, including myself, treat with the lowest, most piddling regard.

~

"Stress."

Like energy, it is so amorphous and below consciousness most of the time, that "stress" is something we "know" is a "problem," but we take almost no meaningful steps to "address." Stress resides in the air quote part of our consciousness, along with other things we "should" do. Even in the alternative world, many people think that to address stress—or even to treat severe cortisol dysregulation—you just do yoga, or go on a retreat, or take some Gaia adrenal herbs, backstroking through a calming pool of lavender and unicorns, and that's that.

But in the functional medicine model, stress is measurable and central. Cortisol, as Dr. Gottfried says, is "the little hinge that swings big doors."

So first, it turns out, you have to test it properly. These tests will continue to evolve, but currently a four-point salivary test or a urine test is done throughout the day to measure how much cortisol you are producing at given points during the day. The test you would do at a regular doctor's office for cortisol is a single blood test—but knowing what we know now about the dysregulatory pattern, you can see that a single blood test is insufficient. You need to see what the pattern looks like *throughout* the day. You need to know where you are on the spectrum of dysregulation.

Then you and a practitioner need to investigate what is causing that stress for you specifically—so you can take the appropriate steps to slowly reverse the cycle. And this does take time, which no one likes to hear. You need to search out all the ways you are pushing the red button—a high-sugar diet, stealth infections, gut infections, food sensitivities, a moldy home, poor sleep, or particularly bad relationships to other people, or to yourself. This is where trauma therapy definitely could play a role. Because if your main stressor is psychological—which it certainly could be—then that is what needs to be addressed. It's just that often a psychological trauma is not the only stress, let alone the primary stress.

And no matter what, you need to keep testing (you know, as with any major illness) to see how you're progressing and to make sure you know when you're getting better. This testing piece is extremely important. You don't want, for example, to stop as soon as you feel a tiny bit better, go join a political campaign with eighteen-hour workdays, only to spiral again into the abyss. (For example.)

Finally, once all underlying factors have been removed or remediated, then you need to *retrain your nervous system*—teaching it to move from defaulting to fight-or-flight mode (the sympathetic nervous system) to defaulting to "rest and digest" mode (the parasympathetic nervous system). This is where all of the things we are familiar with come in—yoga, meditation, acupuncture, brain retraining, tapping, trauma therapy, vagus nerve stimulation, and positive thinking.

But in the functional medicine model that must—*must*—come after you've stabilized the foundation of a blood sugar–stabilizing diet, healed the gut, if necessary, sussed out any infections or heavy metals, and addressed any environmental issues in the home, like mold. You can't meditate yourself out of mercury poisoning.

The tricky bit is, you have to be doing this in a systematic, logical, monitored environment.

That's the issue.

You can't swing from acupuncture to a vegan diet to a paleo diet to a twenty-one-day fast like a wild monkey—while simultaneously drinking loads of whiskey, or still consuming gluten, or still running around trying to achieve huge goals, save the world, save the women, or trying to take care of everyone but yourself.
You have to fully reset.
And you have to do it in the right ways, with a good guide.
Otherwise, the bathtub stopper isn't in place, and you just keep pouring everything—time, energy, herbs, money, hopes, dreams—down the drain.

A familiar story.

And you can see how hard this would be for someone who is already in an incredible amount of pain, not getting the proper care, not believed, and not given any of the right information to help herself. She is in perpetual flight. And as this WOMI spirals down and down and down, the whole thing compounds on itself, because the endless descent into darkness is nothing if not stressful.

It is truly a vicious cycle.

~

The point is, I wrote to Ane, I had read all about this theory, these protocols, and even consulted with one of Dr. Test's practitioners—but we would just have to wait and see what my tests said. They're never what people think they will be. Always, "Nope! You are healthy as a unicorn, Ms. Ramey!"

My tests, I told Ane, had just come back.

Normal levels of cortisol on waking would be between twenty and twenty-five units. Forty would be very high. Fifteen would be low. Ten would be bad. Five would be very, very bad.

Sarah Ramey?

2.6.

Or, as I said to Ane, *two point motherfucking six.*

There is Stage 1, Stage 2, Stages 3a, 3b, 3c, and 3d, and Stage 4, which can be unresolvable.

I was in Stage 4.

Also called "The Walking Dead."

My eyes welled up, and black confetti began to fall from the ceiling.

~

Now, this could all be construed as bad news, I wrote, *but to me, this is great fucking news.*

I was flush with an array of emotions. I felt elated to finally understand. I felt grateful to have a document that said, yes indeed, something is impressively wrong. I felt angry, too. I wanted to bang my fists on the walls, and throw myself out the window of my one-story adobe house. I wanted to toilet-paper the homes of more than a few doctors.

And I felt hopeful. You can only go up from 2.6.

But most important, I felt clear. Obviously things were complex—it is the human body after all—and maybe I would never get better. But I was being *described*, right down to the last detail. I had been seen.

It is impossible to convey the world, the universe, the cosmos of difference this makes.

And it wasn't just Me being seen.

This biomarker, this piece of proof (Oh proof! Sweet, rare, precious proof!), described *all* of us, the WOMI 1s all the way down to the WOMI 5s. It explained how someone so far gone with one of these problems could still have so much in common with someone just starting to get sick.

It was big picture, whole-elephant proof.

And most important of all, this piece of proof explained why this problem couldn't be healed by fighting, or starving yourself, or condemning yourself, or pouring supplements over your head. It couldn't be healed by jogging, or jumping on a trampoline, or doing more and more and more yoga. You can't fight your way out of a stress syndrome. You can't aim healing guns at yourself and expect to succeed. By definition, this problem asks you to relax. By definition, this problem is a *response* syndrome, responding to the aggregate of too much physiologic stress. One researcher at UCLA calls it a "hibernation syndrome"—and as one of the bears in this metaphor, I think this is accurate. It is a very modern illness, and modern medicine has not caught up to it yet. And modern alternative medicine hasn't caught up to it yet, either.

Which is creating a huge problem.

Because if no one believes you, and there are no advanced tests to prove that you are sick, and no practitioners are trained to help you in any meaningful way—and at the same time you have been conditioned to think that you are weak, and in order to prove yourself you need to "battle" your illness—then you are pretty much destined to throw yourself against that invisible wall, again and again and again and again and again, perhaps forever.

~

The moral of the story is, I wrote to Ane, at the end of my very long letter—

Someone should write a book about this.

XO
Scooby

16

And so it came to pass that I learned I was in a kind of endocrine failure.

It was all very *Luke, I am your father.*

Passed down through the generations, from grandmother, to father, and now to me—the endocrinological Force had been with me the whole time.

I became an instant cortisol nerd, and this is when all the pieces started clicking into place.

If you have a cortisol problem, you would be ill-advised to go work for a political campaign. Click.

If you have a cortisol problem, you might want to do yoga—but not *all* the yoga, pushing yourself to be the best, best, best yogi. Click.

If you have a cortisol problem, the last thing you want to do is a three-week fast, or any type of fanatical healing regimen. Click.

If you have a cortisol problem—darling, the harder you push that rock, the harder that rock pushes back on you.

Click.

And of course the issue is not just cortisol.

Cortisol is simply the mascot, the metaphor, the surrogate, the rep.

The deeper issue, the much more serious issue, is *stress*.

Stress defined anew.

Looking at this family of diseases as the aggregate of too much stress, both internal and external, both physical and emotional, over many, many, many years—with the understanding that stress has a real, physiologic, quantifiable, and *cumulative* impact on the body—almost all of the disparate research that exists around these topics starts to make sense.

The literature shows that ongoing stress can damage or change:

Mitochondria, the powerhouse of the cell that produces our cellular energy.

DNA, switching disease genes on or off based on the cellular environment.

Cell receptor sites, making it difficult to get certain basic nutrients like calcium in and out of cells.

The autonomic system.

The immune system.

The microbiome.

The HPA axis.

The brain itself.

All of which we see on full display in a typical WOMI.

And perhaps *most* germane to the WOMI crowd: ongoing, omnidirectional stress (stress defined anew) is strongly associated in the literature with a very important, very recently discovered phenomenon in the brain and the rest of the central nervous system called:

Microglial inflammation.

Micro who?

Please stick with me for just a little more science, and then I promise we'll get back to the story.

Microglia are tiny immune cells—macrophages that surround and protect the brain and the rest of the central nervous system. They are the brain's first line of defense, and become activated and inflamed when they detect a threat.

And what has been demonstrated to activate the microglia?

Ah:

Gut dysbiois has been demonstrated to activate the microglia.
Infections have been demonstrated to activate the microglia.
Moldy homes have been demonstrated to activate the microglia.
Pain has been demonstrated to activate the microglia.
Even emotional stress has been demonstrated to activate the microglia.

That's right: emotional stress can inflame the brain.

That, in and of itself, is a huge finding.
But let's keep going.

The study of microglia is fairly new—for example, neither of my physician parents had ever heard the term until a few years ago—but there is very real research out of the NIH to show that patients with chronic fatigue syndrome and fibromyalgia have been documented to have inflamed microglia—and like any other kind of neuroinflammation, this is likely the source of at least some of the profound fatigue, widespread pain, brain fog, autonomic dysfunction, and cognition issues that this type of patient experiences. A finding that syncs precisely with what chronic fatigue syndrome activists have been shouting from the rooftops for decades—that this disease should be called "myalgic encephalomyelitis" (ME), which literally means pain in the muscles due to inflammation of the brain and spinal cord.

They were right.

In fact, now that we have our terms defined—I, too, am going to refer to it as ME/CFS in this text, henceforth.

There *is* inflammation of the brain and spinal cord in these patients.

Which, in and of itself, should be banner, all-caps, headline news.

Another biomarker! An *inflammatory* biomarker, no less!

Discovered in a large group of patients who are still almost universally considered to be the hysterical architects of their own make-believe disease.

And for me, sitting back and looking at all this data, it now made all the sense in the world that cortisol dysregulation, dysbiosis, neuro-inflammation, dysautonomia, and immune problems would all travel together in an unholy pack.

These phenomena go together because they have the same underlying, ongoing stressors—stressors have all become common-place in the modern world—and that ongoing stress produces real changes in the brain over time. And those changes cause an awful lot of trouble, even though it is all very well intentioned. By producing stress-buffering cortisol and neuroprotective microglia, the body is trying to do the same thing:

It is trying to protect itself.

It is known that if provoked too often, over too long a period of time, and then in comes an additional trauma—microglial cells have been demonstrated to change their behavior. They go into a state of hyperreactivity, or uncontrolled inflammation. That is, once they are primed over a long period of time by different stressors—and then in comes a divorce, a death, a skiing accident, a car accident, an abortion, sexual abuse, Lyme disease, exposure to black mold, Dr. Damaskus—these big *T*'s, in a very specific, genetically susceptible type of person, can switch the primed microglial cells from respond-ing appropriately to responding all the time. And the microglia will actually *keep* responding, even if the antagonist has been removed.

Which should sound familiar to you by now.

Because it's just like the switch from high cortisol to low cortisol.
And it's a lot like the switch from a normal immune response to an autoimmune response.
Or the switch from having a normal histamine response to hav-

ing a constant histamine response (called mast cell activation syndrome—a very common WOMI comorbidity.)

Or the switch from normally opening and closing junctions in the epithelial lining of the gut to junctions in the gut that get stuck in the open position, aka leaky gut syndrome.

Because these are resilient systems.
But not immortal.

Systems that if stressed long enough, break.

Click.

It's not the Lyme *alone* that is so devastating, or the virus, or the accident—it's that they have come barreling in to a system that can no longer withstand the strain. Where a regular patient who does not have these underlying issues would absolutely get better with a standard course of doxycycline for Lyme disease—our WOMI may not. Where a regular patient would not develop a catastrophic fatiguing illness after a car accident—our WOMI absolutely might.

She is predisposed.
She is primed.

Along these lines, I had long known that veterans with posttraumatic stress disorder and Gulf War illness often reported a set of physical issues in addition to the psychological issues. And considering what we know now about the very real, biological fallout of a stress syndrome, this famous suite of symptoms should no longer surprise anyone. They are myalgias, fatigue, brain fog, anxiety, depression, and bowel problems. These are MOMIs, or men of mysterious illnesses. And this isn't some flimsy, anecdotal connection I was hoping would one day be proved correct—the United States Navy itself had already produced research papers documenting severely dysregulated cortisol patterns in their PTSD patients.

The deeper I dug, the more clear it became.

WOMIdom, at the farthest upstream source of the river, is like a modern, multifactorial form of PTSD. But not, *not*, in the traditional ways we think of PTSD or stress. It is a radically incomplete theory to assume that cortisol dysregulation or PTSD or hyperreactive microglial inflammation are driven primarily by psychological distress. That near-universal conclusion that if a WOMI or MOMI's physical symptoms aren't getting better with therapy or medication, it means she or he is weak, or obsessed with illness, or unwilling to take personal responsibility, or crippled by daddy and mommy issues, or just broken—that analysis is lazy, and it's uninformed, and it's mean.

The truth is that the modern world *itself*—from the food system to the overuse of antibiotics to the valorization of stress and sleeplessness—has become a sort of slow-moving trauma.

Click.

Then lastly, deep in the bowels of my stress research, a really important piece came into focus.

In 1995, a large ongoing study was begun called the Adverse Childhood Experience Study, or the ACE Study, which revealed that anyone exposed to trauma, abuse, sexual abuse, or other major adverse experiences in their childhood was up to eight times more likely to develop chronic fatigue syndrome. Eight times greater likelihood is a staggering statistic—and when I first heard about it many years ago, I didn't like where it seemed to be pointing. It seemed to indicate again that the problem is somehow all in the mind.

But in the context of cortisol dysregulation—and in the context of the most up-to-date trauma research—we know that if a trauma goes unmediated (i.e., it is repressed, suppressed with medications, or otherwise unacknowledged), especially in childhood, the HPA axis becomes chronically activated and *does not turn off.* This is called neural dysregulation, or neural embedding. The amygdala and the hippocampus store the traumatic memories and continue to play them—quite unconsciously—in the background, stimulating low levels of the biochemical fight-or-flight response. It's thought to be a protective mechanism—keeping people on guard from ever getting into a situation where they would experience that trauma again. Essentially, a fear pattern becomes locked in the mind, invisibly, and anytime anything remotely triggers that pattern, the red button is pushed. For these people, a continuous (if small) cascade of cortisol and microglial inflammation has probably been happening all their lives.

Thus, another way you might think about this dynamic illness is actually more like a conveyor belt, moving a person through the stages of dysregulation—and that person's position on that conveyor belt is moderated by how many times that individual has tapped the red button.

A high-glycemic diet is going to move a person somewhat down the belt.

Tap, tap.
Lack of sleep will move them a little farther.
Tap, tap, tap.
Developing gut dysbiosis—significantly farther.
Tap, tap, tap, tap, tap, tap, tap.
And if they had a crappy childhood, a molestor, a physical abuser, an emotional abuser, a bad divorce, or a very high-stress childhood:

Tap, tap, tap, tap, tap, tap, tap, tap, tap, tap, tap, tap.

They are rocketed way down the conveyor belt, starting early.
That cliff is going to appear for them well before it appears for everyone else.
Which is exactly what the ACE Study implies, and exactly what you find when you dig into the histories of the severest WOMIs and MOMIs. The number of WOMIs I interviewed who were sexually abused as girls was truly sickening.

So: you're probably not going to become a WOMI if you did not have adverse childhood events—but at the same time, there would be no WOMIdom, if not for the introduction of a high-sugar diet, omnidirectional stress, and especially gut dysbiosis.

But this piece—who gets sick—finally speaks directly to my decade-long standing question that nobody could answer:

Why women?

It's not exactly higher math, but it's not obvious, either. Women's brains—specifically in this case, women's amygdalas—are slightly different from men's brains. The female amygdala is what is called "retentive"—it holds on to emotional memories much longer than the male amygdala. The male amygdala is very responsive with cortisol to immediate physical threat and danger. The female amygdala is more responsive with cortisol to the emotional memories of a physical or psychological threat. The VA reports that women sustain slightly less trauma than men over a lifetime—but develop *double* the rates of PTSD.

This limbic responsiveness to toxic stress is sometimes called having a "hot amygdala." And this hot amygdala has also been found to be the hallmark of another subcategory of human beings, which are:

HSPs, sensitives, and orchid kids.

Click.

There is abundant data to show just how responsive our little amygdala centers are. And retentive.

Hence, a lifetime chorus of "*Jeez, you're so sensitive!*"

We are.

But the similarities between the female brain and the sensitive brain don't stop there. Women and sensitives have another big thing in common: we produce markedly less serotonin. McGill University found that the female naturally synthesizes 55 percent less serotonin in the brain than the male. (Do you not find that to be a shocking statistic? I find that to be a shocking statistic.) And one of the defining genetic characteristics of HSPs is that many of us carry the short serotonin transport gene, the gene that limits the amount of serotonin transported back to the brain. Serotonin problems have long been associated with the mysterious illnesses, which is a more benevolent explanation for the wide use of antidepressants for the WOMI population.

But this easier access to the fear and emotional center, the hair trigger for the red button, knowing what we know now, explains *a lot* about who seems to get sick first. As it relates to the conveyor belt, we always seem to see the same thing:

Women and orchid children first.

If the problem at the most basic level is a variety of unnatural stressors, and then subsequent endocrine and gastrointestinal dysregulation, and then immune dysregulation—women, sensitives, and anyone who has suffered childhood trauma are all naturally a little more prone. Said another way:

Neuroendocrine-immunology is our supercomplicated, not very obvious one ring to rule them all.

And I just need to reiterate, a hot amygdala *would not make you sick* without an additional lifetime of unnatural stress—antibiotics, sugar, lack of sleep, dysbiosis, chemicals, etc.—heaped on top. You have to have both.

And, of course, I had to think about this for a long time.

Because again, it seems to point to the absolute last thing we want to point to, which is any kind of weakness or psychological component.

But that's not what it points to at all.

In fact, that knee-jerk response—that fear of weakness or vulnerability—it could be argued that *that* is the problem in the first place, and the following important distinction (echoing the work of writers like Susan Cain, Dr. Elaine Aron, and Brené Brown) needs to be made, for every woman and every sensitive person across the land:

Sensitivity is not a defect.

To be vulnerable, to feel, is not to be broken or deformed. We just have a slightly different state of normal. If we were defective, natural selection would have gotten rid of us, or the trait, a long time ago. If sensitivity were a mistake, you wouldn't find the same characteristics in every species. Women, obviously, are not a mistake, broken, or deformed—though it is important to understand that up until the turn of the twentieth century, that was the dictionary definition of what most medical doctors, philosophers, theologians, and psychiatrists believed about women. Aristotle and Freud both believed that women were in many ways defective males.

This is highly relevant.

Because what is important to understand—right now, at this moment in history—is that men and women *are* a little bit different (just as sensitives and dandelions are a little bit different), and this sensitive, responsive state of normal has a *vital function*.

Someone on this planet has to stay sensitive to the environment, to our cultural decisions, and to our mistakes. Someone has to be the alarm system for the larger human organism. Someone has to be able to *feel* when something is wrong, if we make the mistake of thinking only logic and science will tell us what is right and what is wrong.

As Dr. Aron says, this is the priestly/priestess function necessary in any society.
The 128-year-olds in 28-year-old bodies.
It is the necessary counterpart to a warrior culture, hyperfocused on dominance and defense.

And in a normal state, our slightly different wiring simply makes us deeply feeling individuals, not necessarily depressive or sick. It makes us artistic, creative, expressive, sensual, and vibrant. Serotonin is the "Don't worry, be happy" hormone. When stress hits, serotonin can be a buffer for this—but without as much serotonin, you do worry, a lot, you're not as happy, and you produce more stress hormones. Unmediated, this can lead to depression and anxiety—but the cause, dears, is not the natural affliction of having less serotonin. The cause is the overload of stress—be it dietary, dysbiotic, toxic, emotional, or traumatic, all of which are in great abundance at the moment.

And that stress is asking to be dealt with, wisely, not suppressed.

Because make no mistake: these illnesses were few and far between before the late 1960s. And it was in the late sixties, and then dramatically increasing in each decade to follow, that we started to make these radical changes to the diet, chemical use, antibiotic use, and the stresses of being constantly connected to technology. And we have not dealt with this wisely. Now, in 2020, we are *way* past the tipping point with these illnesses—illnesses that since the beginning have always affected significantly more women than men. Illnesses with river rafts of fairly predictable symptoms that women have been reporting for decades—reports that have by and large fallen on deaf ears, and earned those women the sole distinction of being difficult patients. A phenomenon with a long and robust history.

But now let's look at this:

On the flip side of all these "deficiencies"—women actually produce much more oxytocin, the bonding hormone, and in times of stress the most therapeutic thing that can be done is what researchers at UCLA call the "tend and befriend" response, the female's secondary response to fight or flight. Our stress response is very well mediated by the megavitamin of other people, especially other women. And this is at least anecdotally true for sensitive men, as well. When we mediate our stress instead of ignoring it or armoring against it, we are driven to create connection and community. And if that isn't beautiful, I don't know what is.

So, right now what we know for sure is that for women and sensitives, when that stress bell is rung too loudly, or too many times without being dealt with, it won't unring. And we have to consider that this is *on purpose*. Our bodies are smart.

A woman may be responding negatively with symptoms and PTSD, yes, but if we look at the causes—rape, abuse, poor diet, no sleep, high stress, bad relationships, and a toxic environment—her response is exactly the right response. Those are bad things that need to be eliminated, avoided, or changed. Those bad things deserve a response, not a blind eye.

She may need to make changes for herself and the way she perceives the world and the stress around her—*or*—there may be something very wrong in her environment. She should feel empowered to look for both.

And this necessary, vigilant, engaged behavior isn't just for the benefit of herself and her own well-being (or the sensitive person's well-being). It's for the benefit of everyone. It is easy to see that we are all on that conveyor belt now. The World Health Organization now cautions that *chronic* illness is a greater threat to developing nations than our old, expected foes like malaria and cholera—a change attributed entirely to the things we are talking about here: a sugar-filled diet, a sedentary life, growing isolation, too many antibiotics, too many chemicals, less and less sleep, and constant stress. All those red-button pushers are part of the fabric of our normal culture, and are only increasing.

This would be a very good explanation for why you see more and more and more patients like me. We are starting to be what is scientifically known as "errrrywhere." These problems are coming to a family near you soon. They probably already have.

And if it has not been made crystal clear yet: *you do not want these problems.*

The sensitives, those lionhearted canaries, have been correctly warning everyone the whole time.

Women have been correctly warning everyone the whole time.

And the female body is totally correct in doing this.
We do not want a highly antigenic, inflamed world.

We would do well to listen to the female body.

Because if the environment is poor, and her intuition has been silenced and shamed, you'd better believe her body is going to be the fail-safe, the bell that won't unring. The invader is *not* long since gone, and in medicine they will continue to miss the point and exacerbate the problem—to catastrophic effect—if they think their only work is to silence the bell.

Click.

17

So.

Big epiphany!

Big, totally relevant, personally resonant, profoundly explanatory epiphany.

This felt like another fantastic opportunity in my life to have the orchestra swell, to cue the red velvet curtain, and to prepare once and for all for a big, satisfying Happily Ever After.

Alas.

~

So, what did happen? What happened after I discovered the one ring to rule them all?

Well, like a good hobbit, I tried to destroy it in the fires of Mount Doom.

I immediately hired one of Dr. Tests's satellite practitioners, a young man who had just begun helping people retrain their HPA axes. It seemed clear that this was my missing strategy, he had a protocol for doing it, and I was ready to get started immediately. This practitioner was very young, and very new to the field, and while I suppose this could have been a red flag, he was knowledgeable and

I liked him. He took an extensive patient history, and he was kind and compassionate and patient. We tested my stool and found, as usual, an overabundance of candida, and, finally, none of my old red-herring-friend *Strongyloides*. We also retested my cortisol levels, and, of course, found them to be shockingly low. And so he concluded that while the candida needed to be treated, the main therapeutic piece missing from everything I had tried before was a controlled attempt to retrain the brain to start producing the right amounts of cortisol and other stress hormones, at the right times. There would be no way to help heal my gut if my cortisol was so low. And there would be no way to curb my other problems if my gut was such a mess. The HPA axis *needed* to be retrained—but not with thoughts, he said. With hormones. It made all the sense in the world to me that we would need to stimulate this system in certain, rhythmic ways to retrain it back into normal functioning—and so I got started with enthusiasm. He put me on a program of adaptogens (herbs to help stimulate the adrenals), supplements to help me quickly detox, and a regimen of potent sublingual hormones, to be taken at specific times of day to help kick-start the brain into remembering its old pattern.

And?

Oh reader.

I suppose you are not expecting that *after* we treated my eureka-epiphany condition of very low cortisol, some of the main features of my life swiftly became:

A wheelchair.
Round-the-clock nursing.
A written will.

Ever the cautionary tale: within a week of starting the intensive treatment, I had what's called an Addisonian crisis (deadly low levels of cortisol) and became almost entirely nonfunctional. Overnight my body went slack, and it became difficult to sit up or stand or keep my eyes open at all. It was as if somebody had cut the power and the entire grid went down.

Up, it turns out, is not the only place you can go after 2.6.

Coming in guns a-blazing, it turns out, with hormones and adrenal stimulants in a WOMI 4 or 5 can actually cause a massive ME/CFS crash. No one is exactly sure why this happens, and it is just an asterisk (if mentioned at all) in most treatment manuals regarding HPA axis retraining. It turns out there is a special protocol for people at the far end of the WOMI Continuum when it comes to retraining the HPA axis, and it is gentle and *extremely* gradual in its application.

The practitioner and I had both missed that asterisk.

And so what we did nearly killed me.

I suffered a tremendous, tremendous collapse, and I could not sit up for three months. My mother had to get on a plane overnight and come live with me again—because I was too weak to be put on a plane to go to her. My practitioner was horrified, and too much of a newbie to know what to do.

So my mother took me to see a battery of local doctors, who of course also had no idea what was wrong, or what to do. They put me on supplemental cortisone, because they didn't understand the problem either, and, of course, those synthetic hormones caused me to crash even deeper. We had to set up a nest of blankets in the bathroom during the day because I couldn't sprint back and forth to the toilet as usual. I lay with my face on a pillow, curled at the base of the toilet, shivering on the white tiles, watching drool roll down onto the floor. Every breath felt like a deliberate effort, and I passed in and out of consciousness all day. My chest was burning and my heart was pounding so hard, I felt it would rip from my chest and leave my body limp, splayed on my blanket in the bathroom. In eleven years, through extreme pain and illness, I had never thought I was actually going to die, even if I often wanted to—but now the clear, cold message broadcast from all of my cells was death. It was difficult to lift my arms or even my eyelids. I could not read and could not talk on the phone. My entire body lit up with pain, as if it were on fire—muscles, bones, spine, vagina—much worse than before, and I could not walk very far without assistance.

If you've ever made fun of someone with chronic fatigue syndrome, with your own strong emphasis on the air quotes, this is exactly what it can be like for many of the severe cases, sometimes even worse, sometimes for fifteen years. I suggest you cut it out with those jokes, effective immediately.

I myself felt suddenly lucky that up until then, I had at least been the Walking dead.

Well? I thought, staring at the bathroom wall.

Shit.

~

This heartbreaking, undead state lasted for two long years.

Every day, exactly the same. Wake, twenty-six burning, liquid bowel movements, sleep. Severe pain, severe gastritis, severe aching all over. Bed, bathroom, bed, bathroom, bed, bathroom. Repeat.

We called Dr. Wonderful, who was very sorry to hear what had happened, and very sorry to hear that I had gone rogue from her gentle program. She made some calls to get me in to the esteemed Mayo Clinic, a few hours away, in Phoenix. Obviously, it was time to bring in the big dogs.

One of the reasons I had never been to the clinic before was that my doctors had always been Mayo-caliber to begin with, not to mention that it's very expensive to travel and stay there while they evaluate you. But the reason people with impossible cases do travel from all around the world to be seen there is that they bring in a team of specialists all at the same time to analyze your case as a unit—which sounded pretty good at this point, and far superior to my normal medical experience bouncing from one doctor to the next.

However, when I was finally wheeled in, we were informed that the Phoenix Mayo Clinic had recently changed its policy and would no longer be bringing in a SWAT team of specialists all at the same time to evaluate tough cases. Instead, it had switched to the more usual model of having the patient make an appointment with one specialist, then wait a month for an appointment with the next specialist, then be sent to three more specialists, with a significant wait time between each one.

Another disappointment. But what else was I going to do? We were already there.

A long string of appointments was set up, and the next six months would be spent driving me two hours to, and two hours back from the Mayo Clinic, wheeling me from one specialist to the next. It's not what we had signed up for, but it seemed better than nothing.

~

First up was a gastroenterologist, a round woman with short, spiked hair and a leonine air of medical royalty. Every sentence she dispersed seemed to be followed by an implied "You're welcome."

But she did listen to my case for well over an hour. I laid it all out, and was grateful for the time she took to show interest, ask questions, and take copious notes. She wanted me to see several more specialists, repeat all the motility tests I had already done (more radioactive eggs, defecographies, barium enemas, scopes, probes, and scans). I was reluctant to put myself through painful tests I had already done many times already—but more important, I wanted to hear her thoughts on an explanation for it all—the gigantic collapse I had recently experienced, the crippling fatigue, the severe aching, the severe bowel paralysis—what could be causing all of this to happen? She gave a reluctant nod to the loose diagnoses we already knew—ME/CFS, fibromyalgia, multiple chemical sensitivity, POTS, a severe pain syndrome, vulvodynia, and a severe motility disorder— but offered no deeper exploration of *why* this was happening, or what the root of it all could be.

And when I started to speak up about adrenals and gut flora, she sternly interrupted me and told me to stop Googling my illness. A look of understanding passed over her face—ah, *this* kind of patient—and she took some time to make sure I understood that all that nonsense and hype about dysbiosis, leaky gut, congested liver pathways, and adrenal exhaustion were not real. Sure, I could pay attention to nutrition if I wanted to—it couldn't hurt—but beyond that, I needed to rein myself in from the fringes.

Instead, she suggested a different, more advanced approach:

A combination of antidepressants and birth-control pills to suppress the symptoms.

Followed by plans to develop a more positive attitude, and better posture on the toilet.

She was particularly interested in my toilet posture, and demonstrated to me how to pretend I was a marionette, with a string coming out the top of my head, and when I sat on the toilet, I was to imagine a puppeteer pulling up on that string, straightening my spine. "That could make a *big* difference," she said, looking down at me knowingly from her erect, tutorial position. As if the real root cause—for all those syndromes, for all those years—was my posture on the toilet.

I sat there dumbfounded.

I hadn't been to a top-tier traditional doctor in a long time, and in the interim I had learned so much about illnesses like mine—real data, good data, thousands of scientific papers on leaky gut, cortisol dysregulation, diet, the microbiome, microglia—that I actually assumed things would have changed in the medical establishment by now.

That was not so. That was not even a little bit so.

It was exactly the same as it had been when I started a decade earlier as a scared senior in college.

And so I found myself scrambling, trying not to cry, trying to convince her to really look at my case history and think deeply about the Why of it all, trying to make sure that our money and time and energy spent getting there were not a complete waste. Did she have any suggestions besides antidepressants and birth-control pills? Besides thinking nice thoughts? Besides sitting up straight?

But aside from being referred to more specialists and repeating the painful tests I had already done multiple times, the answer was:

Not really, no.

And following this, we did go to see each of those specialists she recommended, and their reactions were all roughly the same. When I mentioned to the infectious disease doctor how much better I always got on the antifungal medication Diflucan—something that seemed like an obvious, important data point—he rolled his eyes with some drama and gave a long speech about the kind of people who go in for all that candida nonsense. He explained my experience had been the placebo effect, and under no circumstance would he prescribe it for me.

When I went to see the renowned urologic surgeon, in my desperation, I asked him to take a look at my extremely swollen, bright red left labia—one of my only external markers of something being wrong, my one irrefutable claim on reality.

Side note: you know you're in a bad spot when the only way you have to make people take you seriously is your big, red, swollen labia.

Anyway, this new doctor was sort of the quintessential silver-haired man of dispassionate logic and reason—and I had already been to see him once. And like everyone else, he had not known what to make of my case and had referred me down the line. But several days after my initial visit, I called him again to discuss the labia specifically (as one does), which was at that very moment going through its bizarre, cyclical swelling. It was a Friday when we phoned, and a younger on-call physician had taken the call—a nice young woman, who listened to the situation and agreed that while I was in Phoenix, it would probably be wise to do a labial biopsy, which would obviously need to be done under anesthesia, given the extreme nature of the pain.

They could also do a manual exam and a transvaginal sonogram while I was out, things I had been asking for for quite a while. I was unable to tolerate those exams without anesthesia, and so no one would ever perform them for me—but since I was going to be out, it would be the perfect time to take a look. This sounded like a good plan.

Then when we came in Monday morning, we were surprised to find that the silver-haired doctor was not happy to see us. Not at all. In fact, now that I had returned after he had already said he didn't know what to do about my case, he seemed to have transformed from a once-dispassionate physician of some renown, Dr. Jekyll if you will, to a very different man—a urogynocologic Mr. Hyde. And apparently, Mr. Hyde did not like that the junior physician had put me back into his schedule without consulting him, and he made clear to my mother and me that the hoops I wanted him to jump through for my labia were a major waste of his time.

But, since we were there, in the office, and had been waiting for two hours, he very begrudgingly had me undress and get into the stirrups anyway, frowning as he looked at my labia, which was indeed very swollen.

"Do you know why it's so swollen?" I asked, craning my neck to see him over the paper blanket.

"No idea," he said, almost bored.

"Have you ever seen anything like that?"

"Nope."

"So . . . do you know what I should do?"

He looked up from between my legs and said:

"I would stop worrying about it so much."

The fluorescent lights glared, and the nurse locked her eyes on her shoes.

Sighing, Mr. Hyde said that if I was dead set on it, he could biopsy the thing.

And I was a little confused. This was precisely the reason I had come in—to have the mysterious labia biopsied under general anesthesia. Yes, I said. Let's do that.

"Fine. But I have to do it right here."

My blood ran cold.

Biopsy it right here? But the whole point was that I had a syndrome that caused unspeakable pain at the lightest touch, in the most sensitive part of the body, which was clearly swollen and inflamed. Hadn't we agreed to anesthesia?

But Hyde fixed me with a look of such naked disgust, I felt afraid. He looked up at the large, ticking clock on the wall and told me he didn't have time to take me to the operating room for something so trivial. I could toughen up and have the biopsy done right there with a local anesthetic, or I could leave. It was my choice.

I looked at my mother, who looked like she was going to cry.

What is even happening here? I thought.

Why wasn't this man acknowledging that we had come all the way to Phoenix because I couldn't sit in a chair, wear pants, have sex, or even have a gentle breeze on my vagina without fiery pain? Why was he suggesting *cutting into* that very same aggrieved vagina while I was wide awake? And why did he seem . . . so, so, so pissed off at me?

It's hard to describe the vulnerability one feels, legs spread, feet in the air, three fully clothed people looking down at you, awaiting your decision re: biopsied labia.

"Okay," I said uncertainly, deciding I needed to toughen up.

And thus the plan was set in motion.

My mother was asked to leave, though she clearly didn't want to. The nurse got out a tray of long metal instruments.

Mr. Hyde took out a long needle filled with lidocaine, set his jaw, told me to stay calm, and inserted it into my bright red, swollen left labia minora.

Not since Dr. Damaskus had I felt such blinding, primal pain.

I screamed so loud, the nurse had to hold my shoulders down. The surgeon pressed his eyes shut. He looked exasperated. I began to cry.

"Wait here for ten minutes," he said, "and then we'll test to see if it's numb."
He walked out, and I waited, sobbing in the tilted chair.
He came back in, poked it to see if it was numb.
I screamed.
It was not numb.

Sighing, he inserted the long needle into my bright red, swollen left labia minora again, and injected the lidocaine again.

I was screaming as if my own child were being murdered.
I could hear my mother standing outside the room, sobbing.

He poked it again, and I could still very much feel the touch and the pain—this being the whole point, that my sensation in that area was outrageously upregulated, and not by choice—but he declared that just wasn't possible, that there was no way I could feel anything anymore, told me to try to be quiet, and proceeded to start cutting into my labia.

I have never cried so hard in my life.
And throughout the procedure, Mr. Hyde would not look me in the eye.
He scooped three oozing red samples onto three glass plates for the laboratory.
Then without saying a word, he cauterized the wound.

And when he was finally done, he simply walked out of the room.

The fluorescent lights buzzed.
The large clock ticked.
The nurse put her hand on my arm.

"I'm so sorry," she said quietly.

She asked if I would like Percocet or Vicodin, and I told her I couldn't take either. Pain medication often makes me sick to my stomach.

"Sweetie," she said. "For this, you need to take the meds, at least for today."

Okay, I said. Percocet.

I lay on the table, trying to calm my breathing and my body, my mother now sitting on the couch, looking ashen. The nurse came back in a few minutes later with an ice pack in her hand but no medication. She looked at the floor.

She said, eyes fixed firmly on her shoes, that the surgeon had refused to prescribe pain medication for me. She said he had actually left the building already and asked not to be contacted about it anymore.

There was a long pause.

I heard my own hoarse voice asking why he would not give me pain medication—I wasn't even the one who had suggested it. Eyes on shoes, she said that this particular surgeon didn't like to give pain medication to "patients like you."

I blinked.
Pardon?

"Well," she said, "patients with chronic pain can often go to ... great lengths to obtain opioids. We actually see that all the time in the clinic, and while I'm sure that's not you, it's just that, well, you can't be too careful, and, well . . ."

She was still talking, but I could not hear her anymore.

I realized I was trembling and tears were falling down my face. I could not think of a single word to say. All I could think about was what kind of person you would have to be to travel long distances for a vaginal biopsy and cauterization just to score one tablet of Percocet—and that my doctor thought I was that person. I took the ice pack in silence, put it wincingly between my legs, sank into the wheelchair, and turned my face away. I sat there while the nurse spoke to my mother, who had flown into a rage and was crying as well. They kept talking to me, but my eyes had gone vacant.

Finally, seeing there was nothing to be done and that we were making a scene, my mother wheeled me out to the car and we drove back to the hotel in silence.

When we got up to the room, I asked to be left alone.
And when the door closed, I lay down on the ugly, polyester bedspread. And after a minute of stillness, I started to shake with some violence.

I knew there was no way to undo what had just happened.
I knew that, except for my lodging a bureaucratic complaint, the surgeon would never be reprimanded or held accountable.
I also knew that Dr. Jekyll would forget about me, just as I knew that I would never, ever forget Mr. Hyde.
And I knew I needed to talk to someone, but I had become afraid through experience that my circle of family and friends was going to try to tape the corners of my mouth to my ears and force me to try and look on the bright side.
I knew I should try to take deep breaths, but I was gasping and choking on my own staccato lungs, saliva, and tears.
My mind hurtled between outrage with the surgeon, outrage with the positivity-mongers, outrage with myself for allowing it to happen at all, and back around to outrage with myself for being outraged with myself. Making things worse, the ghost of Caroline Myss

and *The Secret* were back, and I couldn't stop thinking . . . is this my fault? Should I have refused the procedure, even though we had traveled hours to have it performed? Should I have tracked him down in the OR and given him what for? Should I be focusing on forgiveness? Or oneness? Or love? Or impermanence? Am I overreacting? Underreacting? Fucking hell. *Did I attract this?*

Finally, I just fell asleep.

For two weeks, every time I went to the bathroom, the urine passing over the wound felt like acid washing through my vagina. And every time I started to cry huge, round tears, I rocked back and forth on the toilet, unable to stop flashing back to all the speculums and fingers and hands that had been shoved inside me over the years, again and again, and again, and again, and again; flashing to the times I had been flipped over to have a man's fingers forced into my anus, again and again; flashing back to Dr. Damaskus's guilty face, Dr. Urethra's red face, Dr. Jekyll's dispassionate face, Mr. Hyde's angry face—a low monologue looping in the background, around and around:

> *This doesn't hurt. It's all in your mind. This is for your own good.*
> *This doesn't hurt. It's all in your mind. This is for your own good.*
> *This doesn't hurt. It's all in your mind. This is for your own good.*

If there had been any question as to whether trauma was playing a role in my life, and probably my illness, there wasn't anymore.

But something had become clear to me.
My problem wasn't war or domestic abuse or rape.
My problem was the medical system itself.

~

We found out a week later that despite the lab report showing the biopsied tissue was indeed found to be acutely inflamed with high eosinophils, the urologic surgeon had barely written anything about his findings or the procedure in my chart. Instead, what he had written was a note indicating (in the chart that would be passed around to all of my doctors) that he suspected I had come to the clinic in search of narcotics.

The whole scenario was relayed to my family, who were horrified.
They did not ask me to look on the bright side.
Instead, they finally seemed to understand:

This was what it had been like the whole time.

18

So.

Let's freeze-frame Sarah again, cauterized on the bed. She doesn't want us around anyway, and now is a good time to take another break to pause and reflect. There is so much happening here in this Mayo Clinic situation that is not just not-unusual, it's plain routine for a WOMI or someone dealing with chronic pain, and especially pelvic pain.

The problem with pain, just like the problem of all invisible illness, is that it requires belief. You can't see it. You can't prove it. You can't get it notarized. You can only circle one of ten cartoon faces on a gradient of happy (1) to frowny (10) on the famously insufficient pain scale. This inability to easily express these crucial facts of your life carves a gulf deep and wide between you and the faraway shores of being Seen and Heard and Understood. And so if the physician sitting opposite you is more of a Dr. House and less of a Marcus Welby—that is, he subscribes to that strongly held belief that logic and reason reign supreme and are only spoilt by the muddying effects of feeling and relationship—you can find yourself in serious trouble. Such doctors simply don't have the capacity or the inclination to feel your pain, and there is quite literally nothing you can do to convince them if they have already decided that the real problem at hand is actually a defect in your personality.

Observe:
The normal human cues we use elsewhere to convey distress seem, in this case, to have the opposite effect on a Gregory House. Especially if you are a woman.

If you cry, a totally natural response in many hostile medical settings, or if you're in a lot of pain, then you can be (and often are) pegged as overemotional and irrational. If you become angry about having a piece of your vagina cut out, you can be labeled as "difficult"—or, in my case, a junkie. And if you are visibly sad or depressed, you can of course expect to be shunted almost immediately into the unhappy company of the overmedicated and heavily sedated. It is a form of control you have no control over. And if this is happening to you, it just makes you even sadder, more angry, and needing to cry.

It is the definition of gaslighting.

Accusing you of being overemotional, while doing the very thing that is making you overemotional.

And over the course of a long illness, the effect on the patient is devastating.

But the bizarre tragedy is: a stark lack of empathy could, and probably should, be considered a serious emotional problem. Especially, I would say, in a physician.

Let's look closer at my example.

There in the office with Mr. Hyde, where my composure fell apart (and whose would not?), my tears seemed to fuel disproportionate levels of disgust, anger, and even tamped-down rage on the other side of the stirrups. Because it is not rational thinking to conclude that a patient would ask to have her vagina cut open in exchange for one tablet of Percocet. It is not rational thinking to conclude a patient has conjured her own swollen labia by the tremendous, supernatural powers of her ability to psychosomatize—and yet some kind of prejudice (Was he antiwoman? Anti-WOMI? Having problems at home? Just an asshole?) was so aggressively a part of this particular surgeon's psychological complex that all his reason and rationale and logic seemed to go straight out the window. Of the two of us—me wailing and him with steam coming out of his ears, stomping around, slamming doors, and fleeing the scene—I'm not sure who would win the contest for "most incapacitated by emotions."

And of course the reason this matters so much is that this scenario has real consequences. In my case, I came to real physical harm, real psychological harm, and I left the clinic much worse than when I got there. We would have to spend many months getting his comments expunged from the record so that they wouldn't wrongly cloud future doctors' perception of me as an opioid junkie. So not only was there harm on all levels and a bit of character assassination—we also had to *pay money* for it. A lot of money. Our Mayo Clinic experience, including the long stays in hotels while waiting for appointments, came to the tune of a staggering twenty thousand dollars.

But for the surgeon, life would just continue as usual.

There is no diagnosis for empathy deficiency, for assholishness, for sexism—especially if it wears a white coat, male or female—and we certainly don't medicate these people, or ostracize them. Come to think of it, we make TV shows about this exact kind of person, and they are not the villains. They're the heroes.

But as a patient, especially if you are very sick with an undiagnosed and invisible problem, this equation, in plain language, sucks. You have nearly no leverage to advocate for yourself, or to fight back. You are there specifically because you are weak. And so if the person with the power abuses that power—if the person in power is operating under the faulty algorithm and believes that pelvic pain, chronic fatigue syndrome, fibromyalgia, irritable bowel syndrome, and the rest of the WOMI masses are different versions of All In The Mind Syndrome or Irritable Woman Syndrome, and if they actually seem to pride themselves on putting these soft-headed ninnies in their place—well then, my friend, you are in a very real bind. You can't wheel after them, yelling obscenities. You can't leave a bag of dog poop on their desk. You can't egg their car. You definitely can't cry or make a fuss. This doesn't do anything except to prove their point—that you are unstable, and unworthy of serious medical attention. In some cases, of course, you can sue, but exactly like sexism, racism and most isms, the offense is usually not blatant, not actual malpractice, and is done behind closed doors. And even if you do sue, that is expensive, emotionally exhausting, and actually stigmatizes *you* as the craven patient, out to make a buck—all things you cannot afford.

This is, if you are wondering, why I had never sued any of these people.

Because it is an impossible situation.
And you need to spend your precious time, energy, and money getting well.
Not fighting a losing battle.
Usually, no one else is there to witness their bad behavior except you, and perhaps the nurse—and the latter may have learned just to look at his or her shoes.

And this is exactly what makes the New Age campaign against the "negative" emotions so destructive. Because negative emotions are sometimes exactly the right emotions.

It's more unsettling if you aren't a little angry when something truly vile has happened. Healthy anger is how we set a boundary, especially when we're dealing with people who are not interested in our boundaries.

This is vital.

Because the truth is, if you don't have that capacity—and if you are not protected in your right to say no, to resist—it is smooth sailing for the Mr. Hydes of the world.

If you don't have that capacity, you have become deactivated.

And so, as in the case of rape, domestic abuse, emotional abuse, sexism, or racism—the invisible maladies of culture—even though the pressure is great to stay silent, even though the shame of being the victim can feel tremendous, even though there may be consequences, this is why it is so important when these terrible things happen to find a way to speak up.

Even the New Agers.
When someone keeps sticking a finger in your eye, you're supposed to say *stop*.
Not *namaste*.

But in the real world, what really happens with the vast majority of us—trauma survivors, rape victims, and victims of sexual abuse—is that we often say nothing at all. Because there are real cultural consequences when we do. And because of this—because of fear of retribution, of shame, of guilt, of stigma, of exhaustion, and just wanting it to all go away—whatever the reason, it is very common just to try to suck it up and carry on.

And unfortunately, that's exactly what I did.

As with every assault that had come before, my response was to swallow the entire experience whole.

If we return to Sarah on the bed, we find a young woman who is clenching her teeth, avoiding her own eyes in the mirror, trying to grow a thicker skin, and pushing herself to be strong and to move on. She wakes up every day, forcing a smile, forcing forgiveness, doing her deep breathing, and determined to heal.

This makes everyone else around her feel better, and she feels at least she can do that. Make everyone else feel better. It is the nice, spiritual thing to do.

But like so many people who decide to take that road, who don't speak up, who don't allow themselves to experience their feelings, or express their feelings in a healthy way, or take appropriate action on their feelings—who try to om, and smile, and meditate away their problems—like these people, we find that when we get down onto that bed and look into Sarah's eyes, the bright light that used to be there even at the very worst of times—sort of a sly, winking kind of cheer:

It's gone.

Like so many people in this situation, her body might still be there going through the motions, and she can still have perfunctory conversations, but Sarah—the real Sarah, the light, bright, ever hopeful Sarah:

Long, long gone.

~

My final visit to the Mayo Clinic was four months later with a neurologist.

After forty-five minutes of deep listening, he decided I might have a condition known as complex regional pain syndrome. He had the appropriate tests run—tilt tables, breath tests, blood pressure tests—all of which easily confirmed this diagnosis.

CRPS, he told us, is considered the most painful pain syndrome that exists.

It ranks at a 42 on the McGill pain scale, compared to the 26 of cancer pain.

The hallmark of the syndrome is something called allodynia, which is extraordinary pain felt even at the lightest touch—something I had been reporting for a very long time. In this syndrome, there is a problem in the central nervous system, and the pain the patients feel is not an exaggeration—they literally feel burning, excruciating pain even at a feather's touch in the affected areas, and it is quite real.

Also, come to find out, CRPS is something of a mystery illness. No one knows exactly the mechanisms of action, and there are no good treatments. Not only that but, for unknown reasons, it is associated in the literature with chronic fatigue syndrome, fibromyalgia, POTS, autonomic dysfunction, and motility disorders. And it usually comes on after a trauma.

It is, in not so many words, Painville of the greater WOMI metropolis.

And most people manifest CRPS in an arm or a leg. But there have been a handful of reported cases in the world of a rather more unfortunate presentation of uro-vago-colo CRPS, and I would be added to that small list.

And how I appreciated receiving this horrible diagnosis.

CRPS (which I promptly took to calling "CRAPS") is real, it's really bad, it has support groups, and it has its own Wikipedia page.

The astronomical level of pain I had been reporting into the void was finally made official, a short eleven years later.

And when I quietly asked the neurologist if you can operate on an area affected by complex regional pain syndrome without general anesthesia or sedation, he stiffened and said:

"No, no. That would be awful."

~

Unfortunately, CRAPS has no treatment.

So as the outer world continued to shuttle me back and forth to clinics and more doctors and more surgeons and more urologists, performing the right actions of worried parents trying to save their daughter again—the actual daughter, the human being sitting in the wheelchair, lying in the stirrups, and otherwise confined to her bed and bathroom, was deathly quiet.

Now that I was the not-walking dead, my options had become rather slim. I could no longer stage a health intervention of my own—no yoga journey, no acupuncture journey, no trip to the Amazon for ayahuasca. Everything from walking to talking made my whole body start to power down like a Dustbuster left too long unplugged from the wall. The doors to those journeys—every single one of them—had all closed.

But lying in my bed, watching the sun go up and down, I still tried to do my daily practice—deep breathing and sending out loving gratitude, gratitude for my relationships, for financial support from my family, for a roof over my head, for sunlight. Gratitude for my constant companion, light of my life, Mathilde. Gratitude for my mother, yet again come to my rescue, administering bone broth and green juice morning and night.

But given the circumstances, deep breathing really hurt, and gratitude felt profoundly hollow. Of course I was grateful for certain things, but my life was an irrefutable shitpile. I wasn't having a tough go of things. I was a collapsed star. I had been hitting deeper and deeper rock bottoms for an unbelievably long time—too long. Almost a decade of forcing myself to face forward, to say *I can do this, I will find a way, I will fight my way out, I will cleanse myself, I will pray, I will fast, I will push, I will try.*

I will, I will, I will.

But now that instinctual will of mine had turned into a definite Won't. I was living in near solitary confinement and had been for some time.

Conversations drained the small amount of energy I had and froze the bowel's meager functionality, so I needed to be left completely and totally alone—bone broth and green juice left in silence on the bedside table.

Every bowel movement was a passage of barbed wire, every nerve in my spine and vagina was on fire, and every cell was blinking Low Battery. I had not seen a single friend in almost a year—I had barely even seen another human being besides my family and my doctors—and there were zero ideas on the table for what treatment we could do that wouldn't kill me or make me worse. I couldn't even sit up long enough to sing a song, my old standby medicine for the soul.

I was alive, but that was pretty much it.

And I had no way to make myself feel better about any of it. I was sure illness had deepened me in many ways, but would it ever stop? How deep did it want me to go? The cosmic gift of illness that people kept telling me about seemed to be a cosmic grave digger—old man Frank—and for no cost at all, old man Frank kept digging my hole deeper, and deeper, and deeper.

~

One morning, after a particularly harrowing night—a night I was so sick, I wrote out a will at 4:00 a.m.—I woke up, and when my eyes blinked open, the first thing that came into focus was a large black cat, sitting on my windowsill, not two feet away from my face, watching me.

Good God, I thought, pulling the blanket over my head. *Message received.*

Things were bad, very, very bad, but I did not need a sign from the gods to know this.

I was in a severe ME/CFS crash, just about as bad as it gets, and I did not know how to get out. Mayo did not know how to get me out. Functional medicine books do not address this dungeon end of the spectrum.

A severe ME/CFS crash, or the very furthest end of the WOMI Continuum, is an almost unspeakably ugly place. Some have to be fed through a feeding tube, some cannot speak at all, and some have died. The isolation is total, and the suffering is relentless. As author Laura Hillenbrand who has ME/CFS, says, "Fatigue is what we experience, but it is what a match is to an atomic bomb."

But for me, the truth was that there was an even deeper problem, and it was not physical.

As the days became months, and the months threatened to become years, and all I could do was look out my window—what I had begun to suffer from, acutely, was a very severe deficit of meaning.

I had lost a way for any of this to make sense.

All humans need this.

I needed something—anything—that I *actually* felt grateful for, something that actually gave me hope, or a path, or a sense of forward movement, or something that felt, in some way, any way, to be true.

I could not tolerate extreme suffering in exchange for the gift of sunlight, Zen as that sounds.

And in the past, this had not been as much of a problem. I had always felt at least some twinge of purpose, some sense of a path, and I had attached a lot of meaning to trying to solve the mystery illness puzzle and save all the women—and in fact I had done a fairly good job, and that puzzle was theoretically and intellectually coming together. But in my own body, that puzzle was still a heap of pieces.

I had attached yet more meaning to my illness-born musical career—the quintessential follow-your-bliss success—beautiful Wolf with red Chanel lipstick, who was now doing remarkably well on the Internet—millions of YouTube views, commercial success, and international acclaim—all of which felt like a distant, detached joke. In reality, beautiful Wolf had moved on from bedridden Sarah, and beautiful Wolf was not coming back.

The way had gone dark.

And so I hid under my blanket for a long time. I had been thinking for days in my darkened room about the Grand Theorem for WOMIs (the neuroendocrine immunologic conveyor belt), and all the various recommended treatments for this modern problem that actually seemed to work—the slowness, the focus on food and the microbiome, the acceptance of trial and error, the focus on personal transformation, and the emphasis on nourishment, both psychological and physical. And I had been thinking about how at odds this approach was to Western medicine, but also to the striving, pushing Westernized alternative medicine practitioners I always found myself working with. And especially how at odds this approach was to my own natural inclinations—which were a contentious mix of the need to nourish and slow down and the unstoppable drive to somehow Win—to triumph over my illness, and over my weakness—to push, and push, and push. And how this absolutely did not work.

Pulling the blanket down below my nose, I stared back at that cat—who was still sitting there, completely still, unblinking, looking right at me.

And in my state of annihilation, with nothing else to do, no distractions, no quest, no light, and a fat, black harbinger parked right in my window—I made a decision. It was one I had resisted for a long time, and one that was not in any way acceptable to my friends and family.

In my mind's eye, I summoned up each dream I was holding on to—visualizing them clear and bright—and then slowly, and deliberately, I started cutting the cord to the rainbow balloon of hope. Not out of despair, but out of need. I knew this was positive-thinking sacrilege, but hanging on to false hope was more painful than just letting go. I needed to accept that there might be no pithy chat with Jon Stewart regarding women's health, and no triumphant return of Wolf Larsen, touring around the country. There really might not be a future, epic husband—not to mention no travel, no career, and almost certainly no children. I was probably not going to save the women, let alone save myself.

Holding on to these bright lights was what everyone wanted me to do, but it felt like holding on to the sun itself. It burned. To me, the time had come to go limp, to fall into the darkness, and to stop thinking about how to get out.

I thought of the poet David Wagoner's words, and closed my eyes.

> *You are surely lost. Stand still.*
> *The forest knows Where you are.*
> *You must let it find you.*

19

Somewhere early on, we had all started referring to this decade of my life as the Healing Journey. People admired me for my determination and courage on my Journey, and told me to stay the course. Stay strong and true to my Journey. They asked for updates on the Journey, and sometimes I appreciated this. Journey certainly sounded better than Nightmare, and being on a path, any path, was better than being lost in the city of woe. I also began to notice that people spoke about this path as if it were mystical—adopting serious, reverent tones when invoking the Healing Journey. I was doing something impressive and aspirational by embarking on this Journey.

And at a certain point, I realized that *Healing Journey* sounded rather like *Hero's Journey*—Joseph Campbell's famous distillation of the one true myth found throughout all cultures—from King Arthur, to Jesus Christ, to Siddhartha, to Odysseus, to Luke Skywalker. It's also called the "monomyth"—the one story to rule them all. And you already know it: it is the There and Back Again story, up the mountain/down the mountain, slay the dragon/save the girl, save the Arkenstone/save the world. It is the heroic initiation story, in which a boy becomes a man, and is reborn into his true self.

And lying in my bed, staring at the wall, for weeks, and then months, and then a whole year, I had started thinking about this story. A lot. The hero's journey shimmers with meaning, which drew me like a moth to the flame.

If you're not familiar with Campbell's work, we can do a little recap here—which you will immediately recognize from the vast majority of superhero movies and most blockbusters:

We always begin with our unsuspecting hero—often a dissat-isfied and restless young man (Luke, Frodo, Harry). Then one day there comes a knock at the door: a hooded mentor (Obi-Wan, Gan-dalf, Dumbledore) who comes bearing a great call to adventure. The hero is told he is the only one who can help tip the scales between good and evil, but hearing this proposition, the hero usually refuses, disbelieving he could be the One. Resistance is futile, however, and soon the adventure has taken on a life of its own—a rapid gather-ing of allies (C-3PO, R2-D2, dwarves, hobbits, Ron, Hermione), and soon a crossing of the threshold into a fantasy, supernatural world. Destiny is now afoot. As they set out, it becomes clear that this jour-ney will be anything but easy—it is a perilous adventure, and the road of trials, ogres, and/or space aliens they encounter will be bru-tal. After many battles of wits and feats of strength, there finally comes the defining moment of the story—entrance into the utmost cavern, where the hero must look death square in the face, ignit-ing an inner fire so hot that it burns away the ego, leaving only the soul, allowing the hero to come into power as the prophesied savior. Campbell calls this stage "the belly of the whale"—the sinking into the primordial mud of existence that both destroys and gives new life. Then and only then—having faced death—is the hero ready to slay the dragon, and protect the kingdom from the outside forces of darkness (the Empire, Sauron, Voldemort). In the process, the boy is changed forever, finally coming into his own—though it is often at a great personal cost. But his sacrifice has saved the many, and it is an extraordinary story of initiation, self-sacrifice, destiny, and valor. It is probably the most beloved, powerful story in the world.

I was desperately in need of a story.

Something, anything, to tell myself to mitigate what appeared to otherwise be an unmitigated disaster.

Furthermore:

Initiation, self-sacrifice, destiny, valor? Why yes, that all seemed like a significantly better deal than a permanent onslaught of ogres, Orcs, urologic surgeons, and suffering for no reason at all. I quite liked the idea of my current situation recast as a proving ground for becoming a hero, a badass, and a caped crusader. In fact, as I thought about it, the book I had been trying to write about my health was very much based on this grand, heroic arc. The whole point was that I was going to overcome the dragon of illness, no matter the cost, no matter the effort, and save all the women.

My answer to this call to adventure, if anyone was wondering (they were not), was an enthusiastic yes.

And so in my infinite stillness, watching the sun go up and the sun go down, I tried on many masks, leggings, and sabers in my mind—Sarah Skywalker, Sherry Potter, Shirley Holmes. I found particular solace in the X-Men—genetic mutants, outcasts, and supersensitive. Wolferine? No, *Vulvarine*. I also quite liked the secret identity set—Bruce Wayne, or Peter Parker. Surely I had already been bitten by the radioactive spider, and soon my heroic talents would emerge?

But in truth, none of it really seemed quite right. Elements of these stories and mine overlapped, but it just wasn't the same. Oh how I wished for Professor X's school for the gifted—an elite training for people just like me—HogWOMIwarts—but instead, I was quite alone, lying in my bed, imprisoned. I considered some of the obscure Greek gods and goddesses like Ariadne and Chiron (mistress of the labyrinth, and the wounded healer), but their stories didn't feel big enough, broad enough. It wasn't that I myself felt big or broad, but my story—and the story that seemed to replicate and connect me to so many others, like so many paper dolls joined hand to hand—that story was very big, and very broad.

That's why I was drawn to the idea of a monomyth—a singular story that defines the human experience. Here I felt more at home—a truly universal story. Something in what was happening to me felt really and truly universal.

But for every hero I examined, only certain pieces fit, and they did not fit well.

For example, what was I to make of the stage Campbell calls "Woman as Temptress"?

Or that I had no real-life mentor at all, and seemed to be on my own to figure it out?

Or that I had allies—but we weren't a band of brothers and sisters on the same journey. My allies were my friends, looking over the edge, watching me from far away—or other WOMIs, suffering down the hall, locked in their own cells.

But the worst disconnect of all was that I absolutely had not slain the dragon.

I could see that so many elements of the heroic story were mine—but my version was clearly going to end in magnificent, humiliating failure. It was as if I was pressed against the mirror, looking through a glass darkly.

And this is how it came to pass, lying in my bed one day—unsuccessfully trying to fit this square mythological peg into the round hole of my life, for hours upon hours (because at that point, I had nothing but hours upon hours)—that it slowly dawned on me:

Perhaps there is a Heroine's Journey?

This thought had quite literally never crossed my mind.

Furrowing my brow, I thought about it, trying to see if I could come up with any examples on my own. I started by going back to Campbell's work—all of which is just brilliant (he is very large-hearted, an empath, and a wonderful storyteller)—but there was a noticeable lack of females in the stories he chose to illustrate the hero's journey. Women and aspects of the feminine appeared more like footnotes here and there. For example, he did say a mother could be considered a heroic figure, as she does sacrifice herself for another, and does undergo a major transformation—and I appreciated this salvo—but comparing Bilbo Baggins to motherhood seemed to me like an awfully big stretch.

Furthermore, Campbell had also suggested that the female's epic role in most of these stories was actually to be the end point, or the goal. The princess, who is guarded by the dragon. M'lady, for whom battles are fought. She exists, he said. She waits, magnetic, inspiring, beautiful—like Penelope—and her noble presence alone fuels the quest. She is the reason. She doesn't need to go on a journey. She is the object, the purpose, the home, and the destination.

And at first blush, this didn't seem like such a bad gig. That concept of the feminine seemed a lot more dignified than woman as hysteric, woman as depressive, or woman as sick.

But at second blush, this magnetic, patient egg—as depicted in the one great myth to rule all myths—seemed pretty . . . boring. She wasn't *doing* anything. She didn't seem to be experiencing anything, except in relation to the well-described hero. Her beauty was well known—as well as her virtue and her goodness. But not her actual life. Not her own individuation and development.

And this train of thought was starting to ring a big, clanging bell.

The personal lives of women are rarely included in history books. The history of medicine is very much the same: women were excluded as practitioners in the medical profession in the United States until 1850, female bodies were excluded from virtually all autopsy and clinical study until the twentieth century, and women were excluded from almost all clinical trials until 1991. (*1991!*)

When it came to a woman's reality—her story, her body, her psyche—errors of omission actually felt the most familiar of all.

Even in the theories of this largehearted empath, whose life's work I deeply respected, I could perceive a veil beginning to materialize, with women and women's experiences hidden behind it.

And importantly: my empath and wonderful storyteller did not seem to be aware of this oversight in his work at all. And more important: *I* hadn't really been aware of it, either, watching and reading and enjoying all those heroic movies and books all my life. I had been content to love Harry Potter and Frodo, and hadn't really thought about wanting more women to fill those roles. But I was beginning to understand that if I were that magnetic, patient egg, I'd be itching to get my big journey on, too. To break free. To live a great and important story.

And so that must be it, I thought.

A Heroine's Journey is just a badass female on the Hero's Journey. Lara Croft, Katniss Everdeen, Wonder Woman, Brienne of Tarth. A hero with breasts, and beauty, and a Valyrian sword of steel. And the reason there were so few examples and it felt so unfamiliar to me was just because women have been restricted, caged, and left out for so long.

I liked this idea very much.

And my television wanted me to like this idea, as well—the female hero was coming into vogue in film and TV, and it was hard not to notice more and more female characters wielding guns, and arrows, and magic lassos, and swords. They were tough and they were strong, they were ruthless, and they were powerful—and it was all very badass and heroic indeed. That's just what I wanted—what I had always wanted. I wanted to be tough. I wanted to be strong. I could accept the initiating fire of my situation if it meant I would emerge on the other side, enemies defeated, ego dissolved, victorious, auburn hair flying wild in the wind.

There was just one problem.

The same problem that seemed to follow me everywhere.

One might call it: the problem of reality.

Because waiting with my mother outside the FedEx office with a urinary tract infection, a runny nose, a distended belly, a paper bag of stool samples in one hand and a large orange container of urine in the other—no matter how much I wanted it, no matter how vividly I could imagine it, I felt pretty sure that the Hero's Journey was not the Journey I was on.

~

I remember this period very well. I was doing that microscopic-steps program to rehabilitate these types of ME/CFS crashes, and I was doing ever so slightly better—but I was still bedridden unless my mother personally helped me to the store, or the doctor, or the post office.

But I was at least able to read again, and so as had ever been my default in impossible situations, I continued my horizontal research. Because now that I had started thinking about myths and archetypes, I really couldn't stop thinking about them.

Something mystic *did* tremble below the surface. I was positive of this. I could feel the reverberations far beyond my own experience—that same tingle we feel when we put on *Star Wars*, or watch the red train puffing out of King's Cross on its way to Hogwarts—symbols and patterns that set off a primal tuning fork that vibrates right down to the unconscious core—the stunned look of wonder on a seven-year-old's face when he watches Luke use the Force for the first time, and that unmistakable feeling in the gut saying, *That's me.*

I could feel that same tremor, but at a lower register.
A slow, oscillating sound.

I already knew that my story was not my story alone—my "unique" story was at least fifty million WOMI strong, and our story also mirrored the story of *anyone* with illness, especially chronic illness—the reversal of what you know to be good and true in the world, the quest without a compass, without a mentor, without allies, and the terrible isolation, the physical prison, the disbelief, and the despair. There was a huge story at play here. Similar in scope, but fundamentally different from the hero's myth.

The more I thought about it, our story of illness seemed to mirror the story of anyone and everyone who had fallen down a rabbit hole of any kind.

Of course, I had already used Alice as a motif every time I sat down to write about my life—the perfect motif, playing out all around me without having to force it at all. But as far as mythologies went, Alice was no Skywalker. And Alice wasn't ancient or pancultural or inspiring either. Alice was a bedtime story for little girls.

Still, I couldn't help thinking of the Caterpillar, leaning down, exhaling a rude lungful of vapors as he puts his central question to Alice: "Who . . . *are* . . . you?"

Yes. Who were we?

~

The beginning of an answer arrived one morning on my adobe porch in Arizona. It was a used, dusty, pastel volume I had ordered— the only book I could find that was overtly about the subject, and it did not look promising. It had cost exactly one cent, plus shipping and handling. But it did have the right name: *The Heroine's Journey*.

My expectations were low. It had only a handful of reviews, and anyway, who was Maureen Murdock? Unlike Campbell, she had not been held up as a champion of thought, showered with awards, or assigned in any of my curricula.

But in the course of a few sleepless nights spent reading, underlining, and starring the margins, the veils, one after one, began to float away.

Taking this book from the shelf seemed to trigger a latch, and the bookcase I had been using swiveled into an entirely new room.

Oh Alice, I thought, looking around in wonder. *How I've misjudged you.*

~

The Heroine's Journey, Murdock explains, is not the Hero's Journey.

Obvious, but no one else had mentioned it yet.

The Heroine's Journey, she explained, is not the adventure o'er hill and dale, and it is not the journey of the sky gods. It's not the journey up, out, over, and beyond—and there is no up the mountain/ down the mountain. There is no slaying of dragons. That is the masculine quest, and the masculine initiation. Important, but different. Women can go on this quest, and do, and this can be counted as definite historical progress. (See: cage, see: six thousand years.)

But it is not the feminine initiation.

The Heroine's Journey, the feminine journey, Murdock explains, is the journey *in*. Into the psyche, the body, the shadow, the soul. It is one of the most common themes in the great literature of the ages, but a trip inward is a challenge to dramatize. So the direction we are all familiar with is *down*.

The Heroine's Journey is the voyage into the Underworld.

Persephone, abducted by Hades.
Inanna, diving down through the gates of the shades.
Ishtar, banging at the black gates.
Isis.
Sedna.
Izanami.
La Loba.

Alice.

The heroine is not Luke Skywalker, Jesus Christ, or Siddhartha.

The heroine is the bride of Hell.

And as I lay there reading, I had to shut the book. I turned my head to look in the mirror on the wall—at my gaunt, pale face and shorn hair, at my aching chest moving up and down, and at my burning body pinned to the bed.

I closed my eyes.

Instead of feeling disappointed or sad or afraid—the hairs on the back of my neck were standing up, and the red train began to pull from King's Cross.

~

The Heroine's Journey, I learned, is the story of descent.

You will recognize this theme from just a few paragraphs ago—the deep dive and pivotal moment in the hero's journey, known as "the belly of the whale." The hero is swallowed into the unknown and would appear to have died. And this womb/tomb image is usually the big, climactic moment in the whole hero story. (See: Luke, see: Death Star.)

It is the theme of death and resurrection, of the protagonist or a god—an important theme that predates Christ by many thousands of years.

However, what is less known, is that before Christ, the resurrecter (and often the resurrectee) was a woman.

It is one of the oldest stories in existence. And it is depicted as a journey into a womb/tomb because in most ancient mythologies the great Goddess is consistently represented in just this way—as the great transformer/destroyer. The concept is found in almost every culture as the same recurring image: as Nature herself. The Earth herself. A destructive and life-giving force that was once understood to be natural, divine, and feminine. Mother Earth, Kali, the Black Madonna—they all represent the great, dark force who returns us back to worms and mud, and is also the great seat of life. While all things must return to her in death, no new life is born without her.

And to meet her, you must visit her realm.
That is, go into the womb/tomb of the earth.
That is, go into the Underworld.

But—and this is the most important part—in the mythologies that came before monotheism, the Underworld was not exactly considered Hell. Scary and dark, yes. But filled with screaming, burning, and moaning rapists, liars, adulterers, and gluttons? No. There were parts of the Underworld for those people, but the Underworld was richer in concept than one of simple damnation. It was a place where false identities were burned away, and where the true self was recovered. In Greece, Hades was the place where souls passed to learn their fate—if they would return to the Upper World, or travel to paradise in the Elysian Fields, or suffer eternity in the burning fires of Tartarus. It was much the same in Egypt, where souls were believed to pass through the Underworld to come before Osiris and Isis to learn their fate, after weighing their hearts on a scale before the goddess of truth and justice, the goddess Ma'at. If a heart was too heavy, it dropped into the crocodile's mouth. Too light, and it flew into the eagle's talons.

And while these stories on the surface look like they are about death, in fact to prepare for or act out the descent story is actually an exercise in exploring the shadow, the interior, the unconscious, the heart, the scales—the destruction of the ego, the reassembly of the true self, and regeneration—all while still very much alive.

The books of the dead were books on how to live.

Telling this story again and again emphasized the necessity of an inward gaze, an inner process and passage, an internal reckoning, and especially a willingness to work with dark material. It is the passage—the only passage—of the self through the narrow gate to the soul.

Because most important, these mystery cults *did not demonize the darkness*, as so many modern spiritual paths do. The modern spiritual path is modeled on "up and out"—rising up and out of treacherous emotions, flagellating the sinful body for becoming sick or overweight, and questing for a mind so calm, so quiet, it nearly does not exist. This is very different from these older practices. These older practices embraced and accepted descent and darkness as vital to life itself.

And the lesson for anyone, six thousand years ago or now, is that a person has to pass into the shadowland—throughout life, frequently—in order to continually dissolve what needs to be dissolved, to retrieve what needs to be retrieved, and to strengthen what needs to be strengthened. It can be terrifying to go into these dark places, and it can burn—especially if you have resisted them for a lifetime, and especially without a guide. And for those who do embark on this journey, it genuinely does feel like a kind of death. These huge myths are not whimsical fairy tales, or even tales of adventure.

For example, how does this ancient, archetypal story of stories always begin?

A trauma.
An illness.
A rape.
A death.

Anything that rips away life as you have known it and sends you tumbling down a long and confusing tunnel to the deep. It is painful, lonesome, fecal, and dark.

Sound familiar?

~

The myth of Persephone and Demeter is our most familiar story of descent and return.

In ancient Greece, Demeter was the powerful goddess of fertility and grain, and Persephone was her young daughter. Hades, god of the Underworld, had seen beautiful and innocent Persephone and wanted her for a bride—so he asked Zeus for permission to take her, and permission was granted. Up through a crack in the ground, Hades came riding in a chariot to carry Persephone away, ripping her from the field where she was picking flowers. In most accounts, this scene is depicted as a brutal rape. Her mother was not there to see, but when she discovered Persephone missing, she searched the countryside, weeping and distraught. Finally, an old woman, the sorceress Hecate, was brave enough to give her the terrible news—and learning that her daughter had been willingly given away, Demeter flew into a rage and sent the Upper World into its first barren winter. No crops would grow as long as Persephone was kept from her. This worried Zeus, who had not intended to see the people starve—and so a new deal was struck. Persephone could return to the Upper World as long as she ate nothing from the Underworld, where the rules were clear: to partake of the food of the Underworld meant one must always return. This deal satisfied everyone.

But then just before leaving, Hades offered Persephone a pomegranate, and the young goddess accepted it. She ate three solitary seeds, thereby ensuring that her return to the light would not be permanent. Every year Persephone would descend to rule as the Queen of the Underworld, and every year she would return as the goddess of spring. She would forever be half light, half dark.

And to the modern reader, this might seem like a miserable template for the journey of one's life.

But to the Greeks, the worship of the story of Demeter and Persephone was the oldest and most widespread cult of adoration in all of Greece. This one story predates most of the stories we know from the Greek pantheon by almost *two thousand years*. Every year, processions of initiates came to Eleusis to reenact the descent into the Underworld, to celebrate this process of loss, search, and regeneration. It was the center of worship.

And why?

Because this process of death and renewal is the story of life itself.

It's the story of nature, of the earth.

The most, most basic truth of human life is that it is inherently destructive and creative—inherently dark and light. And embracing this, being interested in the dark—not shutting it out in favor of the light—is critical to life. The pomegranate, in fact, is the Greek symbol of fertility. Broken open, it looks like a woman's womb, filled with seeds. To worship Demeter's loss and Persephone's dark passage was to worship Life.

The story likely grows out of the older stories of Isis and Osiris—Isis, who collected the destroyed pieces of her murdered husband, Osiris, resurrecting him through sex, time, tears, and magic. Isis and Osiris then ruled as partners, protectors, and mediators of the Underworld. And Isis's story likely grows out of an even older story of Inanna, the original descender, the Sumerian Queen of Heaven and Earth who intentionally dove down through the gates of the shades into the Underworld to meet her dark sister, Ereshkigal. Inanna was stripped, torn, and killed by Ereshkigal—and ultimately resurrected, also by Ereshkigal. Like Persephone, Inanna's journey began with just one descent, but it initiated a turning wheel of descents and ascents—for when Inanna returned, she sent down her husband and his sister to rotate shifts in the Underworld in her place.

And if this story of the necessary cycle of death seems a little brutal, it is.

Much like life itself.

Much like all things worthwhile.

Going into the dark material of our own shadows is *not easy*, but it is necessary for a whole, generative, human life.

It is indeed painful, lonesome, fecal, and dark.

But it is also vital, life-giving, necessary, and miraculous.

And as I continued to read and read, it became clear that this process, this story, is not just a small yin dot on the ruling yang fish. Unlike the hero's journey, this is not one station of the quest. The feminine journey is one of *continual*, conscious cycling through darkness into rebirth—learning to see and gather wisdom in the dark, rather than trying to slay the dark.

It is the whole missing yin mirror of the great masculine yang story.

It is the black fish.

A lifetime of journeying into the whale—the belly of the earth, the human body itself, the psyche, and the soul. Again and again and again, sinking into the actual primordial nature of life, and coming back renewed.

For the heroine, the Descent to the Goddess *is* the quest.

~

All the bells and tuning forks were now ringing loudly in my DNA.

It was as if a breach had opened in the ground near to me, and as I peered down I could see countless WOMIs and sensitives and the traumatized—wandering people, lost people, wanting so badly to be of use, to be heroes, to succeed again, to have meaning—but feeling broken and burdensome, feeling no sense of initiation, or purpose, or utility, or meaning at all.

I could see myself looking up, and she could see me looking down.

And she looked just awful.
Translucent, ragged, hunched.
Poor, murdered Moaning Myrtle.

But something else was clear.

Myrtle's problem wasn't something to do with her, some terrible flaw that required being kept in the basement.

Myrtle's problem was that she had been abandoned.

By everyone who refused to listen to her.
By her doctors.
By her positive-thinking gurus.
By her culture.

And especially, by me.

As I looked over the edge, into my own underworld, I could see that this suffering, emotional, vulnerable, moaning thing was the part of me that I had locked tightly away in favor of my heroics, in favor of my illness slaying, and in favor of my need to save the women. This was the wailing part of me that my stoic wall, my vision board, and my constant cure-questing had cut off. It was the part *everyone* wanted to cut off—to make out as bad, and wrong, and weak. It was the part of me, the failed illness slayer, of whom I was deeply ashamed and wanted to hide away from the world.

And so it followed that she wasn't bravely striding through an old, familiar tale of the Underworld, doing all the right, courageous things in that place of regeneration, realignment, and rebirth. It followed she wasn't embodying the story that had been told to her so many times around the campfire, at bedtime, in books, and in critically acclaimed dramas—because unlike the stories of Luke Skywalker and his thousand Hollywood replicas, stories about the Underworld and the female initiation had *not* been told around the campfire, or in popular books, or in any critically acclaimed dramas.

In fact, this creature's problem was rather clear:

She was completely storyless.
She was completely without a familiar narrative arc of her own.

And as I looked down at her with an aching heart, it was starting to occur to me all at once:

To be storyless is quite similar to being nameless.
A problem I was already very familiar with.

And likewise, it is a problem that seems almost facile and unimportant on its face—but in real life, being storyless and nameless causes real, measurable damage in a person's life.

It's the reason people rightly care so much about representation in popular culture.

We are a species of story.

We require it, the way we require food and water and shelter and air. Stories live at the core of how we construct our identity, our usefulness, our path, our purpose. Metaphors, dramas, morals, lessons—repeated over and over again—we don't just do this for art's sake; we do it for our sake. We need it. And we need *others* to understand our story, without having to tell it ourselves over and over again.

So I kept reading, book by book, and came to find that the story of the Underworld had become demonized a long time ago—not coincidentally along with women themselves and many aspects of femininity—especially women's sexuality, women's cyclicality, women's sensuality, and the full expression of women's emotions (not just the nice, serviceable ones). All of it was cast into Hell—along with the initiating story itself—branded with sin, guilt, shame, and punishment. The darkness had become a place we should not go—where no one should go—and if you did, it should only be on a journey to find those loathsome aspects of yourself, in order to battle, crucify, and destroy those inner demons.

Thinking about the positivity quest so often recommended to me at spiritual gunpoint—this sounded too, too familiar.

And as I lay under my burial mound of books and articles, I drank in these deeply female stories of diving down into the darkness and into the shadow—of *connecting to the darkness*, including your own, not killing it off. About being destroyed, totally, and fiercely rising back up again.

I began to send down bucket after bucket of fortifying female literature to my simpering, shivering underself, because, come to find, a *lot* of women had already written about the female underworld initiation—extensively, exhaustively—but somehow their work had ended up relegated to the dusty, unread shelves of the Women's Issues sections tucked in the farthest, most untraveled corners of used-book stores. But by the grace of the Amazon app on my phone, I could summon these used books from their slumbering shelves, and I read and I read. Because as I did, I wasn't just being educated—I could *physically* perceive a connection beginning to reforge between upperself and underself, deep in my spine—T1,

T2, L5, L6—straightening and strengthening and pulling me out of the fetal position.

The mess of my life, and all that had happened, was slowly assuming a definite shape, a theme, and a color palette—with a beginning, middle, and end.

It was startlingly familiar.

Loss, search, return.
Descent, mystery, ascent.
Destruction, gathering, rebirth.

Jarringly, cellularly familiar.

Loss: the abduction, the confusion, the underworld, the procession of mostly females, the total dissolution of the false self, the futility of struggle, and the abject uselessness of trying to slay anything. This deeply human phenomenon can be understood as a marked separation from, or injury to, the soul—a break that can be initiated by one's own actions, but is more often initiated by external factors like rape, trauma, illness, violence, and systems of oppression. It is the story of *all trauma*. Indeed, if you are reading this and have experienced severe non-WOMI discrimination in your life, you might very well be thinking, *Welcome to the fucking club.*

And the first stage of any trauma usually looks the same for all of us: a freefall into a world where everything and everyone is suddenly upside down.

Alice, down the rabbit hole.

But because we don't teach our kids many underworld survival tips: for a lot of people, this is where the journey ends.

Which is, indeed, hell.

But for others, this initial stage of falling, falling, falling will then be followed by the Search: slowly sifting through the rubble, through information, through literature, through the psyche, through the self. And this work is *hard*. And *slow*. It is the dogged gathering of lost bones, lost wisdom, and the lost self—the search for that which has become hidden, veiled, or cut off. First and foremost, it is a search within oneself—but it's also a search within the interior of the whole, or the psyche of the culture. Because sometimes in our questing aboveground, we lose ourselves. Sometimes the whole culture loses itself. And it has to be someone's job to go into the shadow and get it back.

Archaeology, excavation, and exploration—it is detective work.

Nancy, on the case.

And then finally, with a few vital preconditions, there will come the Return—but this return is different from what we are taught to expect—that is, the princess being saved or the monster being killed. A heroine's resurrection is not a release from the wheel—not an ascension, an end of samsara, a rising out of the body, a final deliverance. It's not a slaying of anything, of bad guys, or dragons, or Orcs, or ogres—not even a slaying of inner demons. A heroine's resurrection is down, *into* the wheel of life—a *rooting* into the dark, turning earth. A claiming of the body, a realignment with the psyche, and a partnership with the dark, wormy dirt itself. She becomes literally grounded. Her whole job is to learn how to work *with* life—including the demons and the darkness—not against it, not transcending it, not denying it, not dominating it, not submerging the ugly parts, not striving forever to be better, lighter, brighter, perfect, best, champion.

Her job is to *understand* the shadow.

And when this initiate comes back to the upper world, instead of that being the end of the adventure, it's actually the beginning.

That person now has the job of accompanying others, guiding others, strengthening others as they go through their own difficult, painful descents, disintegrations, and reconfigurations.

Like Persephone.
Goddess of the seasons.

Put another way:

It is an *ecological* initiation.

It's not about learning how to win or dominate something or someone else. It is about learning how to grow strong roots, and to thrive in connection, cyclically, with everything else.

And this requires not being afraid of the dark.
It requires working with life *as it is*—worms and all.

And as I looked at this, and looked at everyone I knew who had been sucked into the underworld, I knew this was exactly correct. This was exactly what I had seen happening through all those composted individuals I had met along the way, and it was exactly what was happening through me.

Destroyed by illness, these folks generally do not come back as avengers—they come back as health coaches, nutritionists, writers, therapists, activists, organizers, yoga teachers, and health practitioners. They're not warriors. They help people come *down*, down into their bodies, down to the real food of the earth, and down into their emotions, and down into the realities of life—winter and all. Indeed, every WOMI, MOMI, and HOMI I know who has emerged successfully from the chrysalis does just that. Male or female. They give up their soul-dead jobs on Wall Street to start urban farms, or transition their practices of medicine from the traditional model to an integrative model that includes food and rest and herbs. They become guides through the underworld. They come back and start helping people and communities to connect back to the earth and to the body and to regrow. They help people put themselves back together. It is a pattern as predictable, and mappable, as any adventure o'er hill and dale.

And so, in other words, and in a thousand different ways:
The heroine is a *healer*.

Ah.
Aha.
Of course.

Not in a mystical kind of way. It's much more common than that. Just as there must always be someone to protect and defend our countries and our families—the common soldier, who needs a kind of tough exoskeleton to do the job—there must also be someone, a healer, who protects and defends our insides, our interior—and this person needs sensitivity, empathy, flexibility, and a great capacity to feel, without becoming undone. We need these people. While there may always be some kind of necessary deconstruction requiring all the king's horses and all the king's men, there must also be someone who puts Humpty back together again.

And that person's story is dark, cyclical, and feminine.

And just to clarify: it is important to understand that there have also been many, many male heroines. It's just confusing, because we call them heroes. Traumatized—by any kind of discrimination—they are then sent on a long search in the dark, only to come back as fierce community organizers, advocates for the vulnerable, luminaries and lamplighters, helping people to examine themselves, and change themselves, connect to one another as a group, and change the culture. The LGBTQ community. The AIDS community. The Black Lives Matter movement. DREAMers. All civil rights activists. All disability advocates. All advocates for survivors of rape and domestic abuse. Veterans with PTSD who seek help, and then support other veterans with PTSD in doing the same.

We are surrounded by heroines.
And their work is critical.

But they use no swords, no guns, no war.

Because for problems that are systemic, there is no Sauron, no Smaug, no singular villain.

For problems that are systemic, what is required is to walk right into the darkness, right down to the roots, to look around without being undone by fear, and without killing everything off, and instead slowly bringing what is true—even if it's ugly—back up and into the light.

Which is very different from viewing all darkness as an adversary.

No culture can survive without this kind of work, this kind of partnership, and this kind of respect for the shadow and the night. This feminine initiation is as much needed as the masculine initiation. Nothing grows without a relationship with the fertile void, decomposition, the root system, the creepy crawlies, the biome, the bowels. Traditional Chinese medicine doesn't call the bowel "the Mother" for nothing. This is the system that nourishes everything, and it isn't pretty, pink, girlie, or nice. In addition to life-giving, it is also dissolving, disintegrating, digestive, and can be very ugly when it is not getting what it needs. One ignores the Mother at their own peril.

And what a gift it was to me to understand this.

To see that being called down into the bowels of the earth, or the bowels of your life—or literally into your own bowels—is to be called down to the Mother. To see that the person sucked into hell isn't enduring karmic retribution, but has an opportunity to root deeper into her own nature, which she may have lost. To see that though she is stripped, she is also stripped back down to what is more essential about herself, both the light and the dark. And to see that being sent through the mulcher—by illness, trauma, or loss—is to be sent down into Nature—and into one's own nature—but also into the nature of the culture—and given the opportunity to bear witness to what is there, to adjust it if necessary, and then to realign, reroot, and regrow. And then to help others do the same.

Which is exactly what I had been asked to do—over and over and over again. To get closer and closer to my own underworld. To examine what I needed to let go of. And to hold on to what was grounding, vitalizing, and strengthening.

But also—just as important—to get closer to the lost soul and the lost wisdom of the *culture*. To really look at the fact that something is definitely wrong, and, while highly inconvenient, really does need attention. It really does need to be brought into the light, even if there is no immediate fix.

And when I finally recognized poor, forgotten Myrtle locked under the floorboards, I was actually a bit surprised to find that I didn't want to tap or meditate her away, as I had been trained to do. I wanted to scoop her up, and listen to the rage and the grief and the sadness and the fear. I wanted to feel all of it. I needed to feel all of it. That's what had always guided me in the right direction.

And why?

Because everything Myrtle had to say was *right*.

Something awful *had* happened, to me personally, over and over and over again.
Something awful *was* happening in the environment and the food environment and it was making people sick.
And something strange *had* happened to medicine, and rendered it blind and uncaring to so many problems, including my own.

Grief, rage, sadness, fear—those were the appropriate responses.

As with the traumatized brain, while I ultimately wanted Myrtle to come to peace, the first step was to acknowledge that everything she was saying was essentially correct.

And reader, what a feeling that was.

To think about what was *right* with me, instead of an endless litany of what was wrong with me.

To think that my millionth trip into the underworld might not be because I was a very, very bad girl—but, rather, because no one was listening to me, and no one was actually trying to sit with me and study the problem in any kind of meaningful way. That had been left almost entirely up to me, which was an uncarryable burden. I couldn't pull myself up by my own bootstraps, because I didn't have any boots.

To think that this was the problem the *entire* mystery illness community was struggling with.

And I was able to see that I had indeed been searching for a long time—and I had indeed found some really valuable information about why things had gone so terribly wrong for me and for people like me. But it now occurred to me that even if I never got all the way better, the little candles I had been able to light underground were almost certainly going to light someone else's lamp, and that person would light someone else's—and on and on—and perhaps, if I could just keep doing that, that might actually be enough. Perhaps, in fact, that was all I had been trying to do since day one. Considering how complex, how difficult, and how systemic my problem was, and how complex, how difficult, and how systemic the problem in medicine and the food system and the politics of it all seemed to be, this continual cycling back down into the mud actually seemed rather understandable. Really unfortunate, and really wrong—but understandable. Some complex problems require a lifetime (or more) of cycles to figure out—and thousands of lamplighters, not just one—but each rotation sheds a little more light, and then a little more, and then a little more.

This shift helped me to see something I needed to see:

Perhaps I wasn't a magnificent, humiliating failure after all.

I just wasn't a hero.

Which was, in fact, a relief.

I really was the inverse of Harry Potter.
Just an average, garden-variety Queen of the Dead.

My story wasn't about triumph, it was about accepting the mantle of the underworld worker—which is a lifetime assignment of infinite cycles to keep working on a problem until, one day, it is healed. And that mantle made me feel something else, totally foreign to my body.

It made me feel useful.

Which sounds small—but if you've never been shattered into a thousand pieces, you may not know how important that feeling really is. If you've never been told that you are just a broken, rancorous, emotional glitch in the system—over and over again—you may not know how rare and precious and strengthening a sense of usefulness, of utility—of service—can be.

And I realized I would probably do this job a whole lot better if I stopped dragging around my heavy, useless sword, and laid down my meaningless, borrowed armor.

Because a heroine is no dragon slayer.

Indeed, if she believes that, she may very well slay herself to death.

Instead, male or female, the heroine is the protector of the root system, the interior, the interstitials, the cycles—of the body, the psyche, the soul, the soil—of the cultural body, the cultural psyche, the cultural soul, the cultural soil—of the vast and often invisible systems that nourish, nurture, and support everything, in the dark.

Coming to this conclusion, I closed the book I was reading, and laid it on my chest.

And then waving the smoke from my eyes, smoothing my blue dress, and standing up straight—I turned to the Caterpillar, and I began to tell him exactly who I was.

20

Reader, I will tell you something now:

No cure, no juggler, no miracle pill, no positive thought will ever be worth more to me than the story of my story, the story of our story, the story of the ancient, holy, and important dark.

The missing, magic mirror.

21

For months, I reveled.

I mainlined trauma stories, like a drug.

If my last visit to the Mayo Clinic had smothered my hope light, authors like Marion Woodman, and bell hooks, and Sue Monk Kidd, and Clarissa Pinkola Estés, and Virginia Woolf circled around me, relit the pilot, and opened the gas full throttle.

And there was really no way to miss that every single one of these mentors appearing in the forest with helpful hints about the darkness were women. Usually older women. Wise women. Female tutors, quietly expert in the art of fruitful despair.

But I thought this made a certain amount of sense, because of course the song of trauma might be female. It is the female of the species that has been oppressed, raped, shamed, sold, and demonized for six thousand years—and it is the female of the species that has been considered second-class in virtually every country, in every class, on every continent, and in every age. All marginalized people are shoved into this kind of life, but you might make the argument that to suffer in these ways is to enter into the larger, historically (and in many places contemporaneously) female experience.

However.

It was also clear that the femaleness of this subterranean story-of-stories did not end with the authors who told it, or the protagonists that starred in it, or even the historical precedent set by the thousands, millions, billions of women who had lived it.

As I considered it more, it seemed to me that there was actually something about what you might call a fluency with darkness that women, in my experience, really do possess a bit more than men. That is, an evident and familiar ability to deal with pain, or illness, or emotional upset—without pathologizing it, without othering it, and without shutting it down. In fact, I thought to myself, staring up at the ceiling in my own lightless cell, Isn't that ability to tolerate darkness really the underlying mechanism of something light-sounding, like empathy? Because there is no empathy without embracing pain. Indeed, nonempathic responses, like trying to fix something that can't be fixed, or becoming hyperclinical about an emotional problem that just needs to be heard out, or closing down in the face of someone else's suffering—these are all ways of denying the dark, and staying safe up in light. Empathy is not sweet or sugary or nice—it's about the strength it takes to go down and be with the dark.

In fact, I thought, continuing to mine this seam, there is a very similar process at play for traditionally feminine qualities like compassion, and sensitivity, and inclusion, and self-inquiry, and self-development, and self-care. Contrary to branding, embodying these qualities is not snuggly or cute or dear or darling—embodying these qualities is actually quite hard. Because there is no compassion or inclusion without welcoming other people as whole, both their lightness and their darkness, their sameness and their difference—which is an incredible challenge. Likewise, there is no self-inquiry or self-development or self-care without being willing to look at your own shadow, at what you yourself might be doing that is hurting you or others—which is very hard, internal work. Even a quality like nurture is about the darkness, because there is no real way to nurture yourself (physically) without long, deep sleep, or to nurture someone else (emotionally) without long, deep conversations about the hidden compartments of the heart.

All of these are stereotypically feminine qualities, and all of these stereotypically feminine qualities:

Why, they are quite difficult.

They require real psychological resilience.
They require real emotional intelligence.
They require real temperamental fortitude.

And most important, they require a real willingness to spend time in the dark—and this was such a novel idea for me to begin to wrap my mind around.

Being feminine was not Barbie pink.
Being feminine was deep, blood-red.

And at least in my own life, I really did see those qualities on display more clearly and more often in most of the women I knew, in addition to my gay and HSP male friends—that is, my gay and HSP male friends who were almost universally seen by those around them as markedly more feminine.

Then, when I put all this together with the heroine's story—the epic tale of the Underworld, of the healer, of resilience, of the loud and outspoken activist who speaks up, over and over and over again (sometimes with anger, sometimes with rage) when something is wrong down in the root system—when I looked at things this way, I was beginning to realize (with not a small amount of embarrassment) that being "feminine" looked a lot different from what I somehow believed, perhaps not consciously, not actively, but tucked away and operating on silent in the back of my brain.

But now that it was at the front of my brain, I had a good idea where it had come from.

The feminism I grew up with (and probably the feminism you grew up with) was the type of feminism that worked hard to argue that men and women are Equal, and Equal means the Same. I learned that to be a girl on equal footing with a boy was to be a girl who was bold and assertive, not passive and demurring. To be a girl who was equal to a boy was to be strong and tough, not sensitive and soft. And to be a girl who was equal to a boy was to be ambitious and striving, not lazy or indulgent.

Indeed, this kind of feminism is alive and well today.

And to be sure, women and feminists have worked toward this goal of sameness for very good reasons. "Biology as destiny" has always been used *against* women, and there is a robust history of men maligning women for being too nurturing for the dog-eat-dog world of industry and commerce; for being too compassionate to be an effective soldier, sergeant, general, or commander in chief; and for being too emotional to be an effective and dispassionate CEO. In fact, my famous endocrinologist grandmother's entire career revolved around explaining to the public that women are just as competent as men, biologically, intellectually, and otherwise—because just forty years ago, women being just as competent as men (biologically, intellectually, and otherwise) was absolutely not the reigning ideology.

And so I had grown up subscribing to this idea:
Equal means the Same.

Be bold, not passive.
Be strong, not sensitive.
Be tough, not tender.

And in my mind, this had nothing to do with gender.

I was simply choosing the best qualities one should have.

In fact, I was firmly gender-neutral. The captain of my own ship, the scribe of my own story.

I had internalized the famous academic Judith Butler's idea that gender is a performance, a social construct, a mental construct—and that underneath all our conditioning we are actually all completely gender-fluid and gender-ambidextrous, and therefore we all chart our own course when and if we choose to do so.

I had been choosing to do so, with some verve.

And, to be very clear, this was not some wrongheaded misadventure. Dismantling the old idea that gender dictates how you *must* act and *should* act in certain masculine or feminine ways because of your hormones or your brain—this kind of social deconstruction, this troubling of gender, as Butler would say—really is radical and important work. It helps undo assumptions and stereotypes that can be extremely limiting, insulting, constraining, or just wrong for all of us, but especially for the sizable proportion of each gender that does not conform to gender norms—that is, women who are just naturally more masculine, men who are naturally more feminine, nonbinary people, trans people, queer people, and on and on. That diversity within each gender obviously exists, and should be both accounted for and protected. We should indeed be free to chart our own course, and no one *should* be required or expected to behave one way or the other.

But this good idea overrides another crucial point.

Just because there is diversity within each gender, which there clearly is, does not mean that gender does not exist at all. It does not mean that a majority of women, and a majority of men, cannot and do not exhibit behaviors that *do* correspond to their gender.

And while it is difficult to parse out definitively what is learned versus what is inherent, one thing is very clear, and I will use myself as an example:

As I lay there looking back on my own social performance, I simply could not deny that the *reason* I had primarily distanced myself from being gendered in the first place—the reason I had gone to such lengths to show that gender neutrality was real and important and my own North Star—was not actually because of this good, deconstructive, gender-fluid ideology.

If I were painfully honest, the real reason was:

I was afraid.

I didn't like to think about, or name, or associate with gender, because if I did, as a woman, I might very well be associated with *feminine* qualities.

And I certainly didn't want that.

Aha.

~

Okay, reader.

I know you, and I see you.

Friend, I *am* you.

Your hackles are raised, all the way up to the sky.

Conversations around gender *really* rile people up, my recent self included.

However, we are going to proceed down this fraught path anyway, whether or not you are huffing and puffing—and in order to do so, we have to venture even further into the world of the woo. Because to have this dialogue at all, we need to actively define those mystic qualities currently hovering above and around our discourse, which are:

The Masculine, and the Feminine.

And while I know this surely seems like an unpleasant trip back to the 1950s, please rest assured that in this masculine/feminine conversation we are not talking about women being from Venus and men being from Mars. That is indeed outdated, restrictive, and wrong. There is clearly not a 1:1 ratio of man: masculine, woman: feminine. Obviously not. We all have all of these qualities swirling within us, and we all have the potential to develop these qualities to greater and lesser degrees if we set our minds to it. We are all from Earth.

But the concept of yin and yang is one of the oldest, most universal concepts in existence—so pooh-poohing it out of hand as superstitious nonsense, in my view, is both hubris and a mistake.

Virtually everywhere else in the world, there is a basic understanding that masculine and feminine energies are found in everything in the world around us, from plants to houses to horses to human beings. These energies are considered opposing but complementary forces—which flourish when they are maintained as coequal partners.

And the more I mapped out the properties of each for myself, the more I saw that this was inarguably true.

So hold on to your hackles, because we're going to rip that Band-Aid off now.

~

Masculine energy (yang, the white fish) is classically understood to be:

Linear, logical, goal-oriented, assertive, focused, structured, self-reliant, intellectual, stoic, dispassionate, contained, disciplined, strict, ascetic, outward-focused, ascending, and objective. It is interested in solving and fixing immediate problems, interested in achievement, interested in healthy competition, interested in objective knowledge, interested in physical and intellectual strength, and it views darkness as something wrong and bad to eliminate. It is associated with the sun, daytime, and the upper world. And if a person or a community becomes hypermasculine, the individual or group becomes rigid, dominating, aggressive, overly focused on fixing, perfectionist, sterile, authoritarian, warlike, disconnected, and emotionally shut down.

Then, on the other side of the ledger, we have feminine energy (yin, the black fish), which is classically understood to be:

Cyclical, intuitive, receptive, magnetic, diffusely aware, flowing, relational, soulful, vulnerable, deeply feeling, wild, creative, nurturing, nourishing, inward-focused, grounding, and subjective. Feminine energy is interested in looking at the big picture and the long term, interested in celebrating what has already been achieved, interested in win-win solutions, interested in experiential and embodied knowledge, interested in emotional strength, and views darkness as something to investigate and learn from. It is associated with the moon, nighttime, and the Underworld. And if a person or a community becomes hyperfeminine, things become chaotic, unstructured, raging, unable to make progress, devouring, passively destructive, prone to addiction, prone to victimhood, and emotionally volcanic.

Complementary, but fundamentally opposing.

Even in the negative: if one finds oneself in a hypermasculine situation, one can be sure that a hyperfeminine backlash is not far behind, and vice versa.

See: the USA.

And so the basic idea is that health exists when there is a cultivated balance between the positive sides of both. For example, a robust military *and* a robust social safety net.

But that concept—healthy tension—is where we get into trouble.

Because we don't consider these two ledgers to be coequal, complementary, balancing partners.

We arrange them in a hierarchy.

Masculine *over* feminine.

So if you go back to the idea of gender neutrality and bear that out, pretending we are all just choosing from the very best qualities one can have—well, when you put these two ledgers back-to-back, what you will actually see is that in these "gender-neutral" environments, most of us are actually defaulting to some preference for the masculine, almost all the time.

Logic almost always trumps intuition.

Objective data almost always trumps subjective experience.

Striving almost always trumps self-care.

We love heroes, we don't even know what a heroine is.

That is not neutral.

Go right down the list, one side back-to-back with the other, and you can see it very clearly.

Most people need to be assertive to get ahead, not receptive to new ideas.

Self-reliant, not asking for help.

Outwardly focused, not inwardly focused.

The feminine gets a fair amount of lip service—but it's usually just that, lip service. We all know care is a good thing, compassion is a good thing, and empathy has become a buzzword—but when it comes down to brass tacks, we also all know what side you have to choose in order to get ahead, to get paid, and to be taken seriously.

Which should not be a surprise.

Six thousand years of patriarchy does not just evaporate.

And it is not a shock that the patriarchy created the world in its own image.

But somehow, even as a very active feminist, I had not quite realized this. I was not conscious of any real delineation between masculine and feminine, and so I definitely had not realized that unequal value system was absolutely alive in me.

Since the masculine got all the good words (*bold, assertive, logical, reasonable*) and embracing the feminine, frankly, seemed soft—I had just chosen accordingly. Nurturing, intuitive, empathic—these were okay qualities in their own way, but obviously secondary to bold, assertive, reasonable logic. I knew that trusting my intuition should be kept to myself, my subjective experience was in the end just anecdotal, self-care was an indulgence, being too receptive was passive, asking for help exposed weakness, sensitivity was annoying, inward exploration was naval gazing, and on and on down the list.

And so as I read about the real Heroine's Journey, which was pretty much constructed *entirely* of feminine qualities—and was so simultaneously and utterly badass, inspiring, and necessary—and then as I rethought how valuable and difficult and brave and tough all those feminine qualities really were, contrary to what I had been thinking for pretty much my whole life, I could not help but think to myself:

Shit.

Because that tuning fork was ringing loud and clear again.

This problem, this diminishment of the feminine, wasn't just some big, intangible sociocultural problem Out There.

This problem wasn't just one of many.

This problem was, I realized with some surprise:

The problem.

Not just Out There.
In Here.
All the way in here.
In my body.

In my poor, bedridden, scraggly-haired, gaunt body.

This idea that was slowly coming together for me, like another Magic Eye, was absolutely related to the problems of the mysteriously ill.

Allow me to connect these dots for you in exactly the manner I began to connect them for myself, brow furrowed, lying there in my bed, consuming this mountain of literature, finally from a range of female perspectives, all of them employing a rare but truly feminine gaze.

Ahem:

When we do make this decision—
When we do choose to delegitimize feminine values as silly and unimportant and soft and weak—

When we as a culture choose not to turn off, not to rest, not to cycle, not to value the darkness the way that we value the light—

Well, what, oh what, is the body's most famous first responder?

That's correct, good reader.
It is our old friend and hormone:

Cortisol.

The mascot.

Pushing constantly, whether late into the night at work, or at Acroyoga, or chasing adrenaline on the weekends—which is considered a badge of honor for the tenacious modern person—overrides the need for those "soft" qualities like rest, the need for rejuvenation, and the need for regularly checking in to see how the body is doing.

Then, as you remember: a high-sugar, high-caffeine, high-glycemic diet—often constructed to keep us going even though our bodies feel exhausted and could use some self-care—this doesn't just register as delicious. It registers as stress. Too busy ascending to sleep, make food, or move the body—these are all deficits registered as stressors.

Add to this a chemical makeup regime, to appear bright and sunny and pleasing, all the time.
Add to this a battery of chemical housecleaning products, because organic products are less efficient for the fast-paced, go, go, go life.
Add to this the devices you keep in your purse or your pocket that are designed to keep you On from the moment you wake up to the moment you fall asleep.
Add to this the tyranny of positive psychology trying to keep you happy and grateful and peaceful and smiling, no matter what, no matter how steaming the shitpile of your life.
Add to this a culture of sexual assault and discrimination that simmers below the surface, that is routinely and institutionally disappeared and papered over and made to look as if everything is fine, just fine, nothing to see here.

We have become a people who live increasingly for the solar aspects of our lives. We strive for this at all costs—even if it means burning out, or burning up in the sun. Even if it means airing commercial after commercial for prescription medications that depict happy families running down happy, sunny beaches, while the happy narrator reads off a list of happy-sounding side effects, including but not limited to vomiting, headache, diarrhea, weight gain, somnolence, scaly eyeballs, dementia, worsening depression, suicidal thoughts, and suicidal actions—all read in bright, encouraging tones, as if reading off a list of ice-cream-cone toppings.

It is wrong.

And we all know it.

And none of this behavior is any one person's fault—it's not *your* fault—we are all living in the modern world, keeping pace, and trying to be successful, normal, modern people, and if we slow down, we fear we will be left behind.

But the body, *especially the female body and HSP body* (more on this shortly), does not consent to permanent ascent. And the body will not be shy or demure in the way that she lets you know.

Cortisol becomes dysregulated.
Cortisol hogs cell receptors, and the sex hormones start to dysregulate.
The period becomes a monthly, worried telegram.
The infections begin.
The insomnia sets in.
Energy wanes.
Anxiety soars.
Allergies develop.
Poop becomes an unwanted matter of serious and frequent concern.

We've been over this, just not with our controversial but helpful Masculine/Feminine ledger on hand. But when you look at things through that particular prism, it all begins to make significantly more sense.

If a person has no understanding that she has the absolute right to be feminine, to be sensitive to her underworld's signals—and there are no systems in place to support this right—and if the environment she is living in is a bad one, partly by her own creation, but mostly driven unconsciously by the culture at large—well, then she is going to override this critical message. Instead of going down and in, she will brush her shoulders off and soldier on. She will lock the basement door and lose the key.

And she will be applauded for this. She is leaning in.

But if the environment is unsafe, the endocrine system, the nervous system, and the immune system *do not want the body to fight, toughen up, paper over, or ignore them.* These systems want the person to slow down, drop in, listen, and respond wisely—sooner, not later. Something is wrong in the root system and it needs to be attended to. These signals being sent in the beginning will not kneecap her— they do not want to harm her. They just nag, and pull at her pant cuff. Like emotions, like children, they want and need to be heard.

Thus the sensitive body requires that it be strong in this other, important way—the way that is not valued almost at all—the strength it takes to make time, to be willing to change behavior, to change the environment, and to tell other people that something subtle is wrong and needs tending before it snowballs out of control.

This is wisdom, not weakness.

Yet it is perceived and treated as the exact opposite.

And why?

Why don't we know any better—doctor *or* patient?

Why is it such a radical idea that food and rest might impact our health so greatly, and why is it a dangerous idea to suggest dietary change (which requires some inward analysis, and is also associated with the domain of women, aka food) as a saner starting place before resorting to medication upon medication? Why does it take so, so very long to find out about the actual roots of these problems? Why are the symptoms of early cortisol dysregulation, or any endocrine dysregulation—anxiety, being wired and tired, insomnia, problematic periods, cystic acne, fatigue, bowel problems, frequent infections, allergies, eczema, and an inability to lose weight— universally ignored and deemed unimportant? Why, when it all starts to avalanche into severe bowel problems, severe depression, severe inflammation, severe immune dysregulation and autoimmune disease—why are we still so surprised, claiming the causes are utterly unknown, and all there is to do is take medications and sedatives and antidepressants to keep suppressing the symptoms?

Don't we have the best medical care in the whole world?

Put simply:

No.

Our medicine, put simply, is missing its other half.

The darker half.
The slower half.
The more compassionate half.

The half that is willing to descend, to search and figure out what is truly going on, no matter how inconvenient it is—so the patient can finally, genuinely ascend.

This imbalance, this missing partner, is a big part of the reason our health care system ranks thirty-seventh in the world.

This imbalance is a big part of the reason we excel at acute (heroic, eliminate the bad guy) illness and can't for the life of us solve chronic (heroinic, root system) illness.

This imbalance is the reason when our female protagonist finally goes to the doctor for her mysterious illness, and she reads her Magna Carta of symptoms, possibly breaking into tears because she has been dragging this weight for so long, she can be pretty sure that the white rabbit remedy out of a hat, the maverick solution, is always, always going to be Prozac. Or Lyrica. Or Abilify. The answer is always going to be that she is antidepressant-deficient, Watson.

The answer is quite literally that she should smile more.

Because good doctors—whether they are male or female—abide by masculine expectations, and are only expected (and given time) to slay dragons, shoot at symptoms, kill disease, and surgically remove or fix problems. They don't get trained or paid for much of anything else. And if they critique this at all, suggesting that their field consider things like food and sleep, it will be used against them, pegging them as unserious and too soft.

Similarly, Good Girls don't and won't go to Hades. Good girls strive, no matter the cost. We get good grades, good degrees, we make a difference, we juggle family and work, we swallow our anger, and we prove that women can do anything men can do. And when we realize this doesn't work, and we try to critique this expectation and demand what would actually be better for us—that is, a world made in *our* own image—like a better work-life balance, like more help from men doing traditionally feminine work like child care and house chores, like better food for our families, like makeup that doesn't disrupt our endocrine system, like paid family leave, and like universal day care—this is used against us. Unserious. Too soft. Too much. Indulgent. And then when symptoms do inevitably arise, we are simply told to medicate everything and carry on—and if we can't carry on, and if our problems can't be fixed in fifteen minutes, and especially if we happen to be women, our illness quickly becomes our hypochondria, our depression, our madness.

Reader, it is wrong.

And both entities—the doctors and the good girls—have the same thing in common. We are all severely feminine and underworld-deficient. None of us has any experience working with the roots—which is difficult work, dark work, and work that takes more patience, more compassion, more strength, and more time.

And who has the time?

But it all just produces a never-ending medical Whack-A-Mole.
As soon as any of these symptoms come up, *whack*, we just shove
them back down.
As soon as a difficult patient comes up, *whack*, Cymbalta.
Not my specialty? *Whack*, off to another specialist.
Too many symptoms? *Whack*, it's all in your mind.

It's a comedy for the pharmaceutical companies.
And a tragedy for everyone else.

My good reader, it is monumentally wrong.

But also, when we do this, when we keep this important door
to the underworld locked, when we demonize the feminine in our
bodies, in our lives, in our medical system—when we are not encouraged to embrace any kind of darkness, offness, slowness, any unpretty
symptoms, or anything less than perfection and superwoman or stoic
man, all the time—when there is no time to slow down and respond
to the red flags in our lives, or, for that matter, to the orange, yel-
low, and even green flags—no time to say hello, goodbye, we're late,
we're late, we're late—when we do this, reader, we don't just hurt our
women and our sensitive men.

When we keep this important gate locked, we are doing something else:

When we do this, we are ensuring an arrested development—for
each and every one of us.

Not having an initiation into the difficult passage through our
own interior guarantees an extended age of adolescence, and one
struggles to find a more apt descriptor of our culture at this particular moment in history.

And yet, I must tell you, something else seemed quite clear to me,
lying there in my bed, thinking about all I had gone through, what all

the WOMIs I knew were going through, what *all* the abductees into the underworld learn whether they like it or not:

Adolescence must come to an end.

If not by choice, eventually by force.

And that is exactly what is starting to happen.

Because in a deeply unbalanced state—where only the logical mind is valued, where only striving and achievement are valued, when the lights never turn off, when the seasons don't matter, when symptoms are repressed instead of understood, when empathy is uncommon, and when the algorithm trumps the story—this is when the need for the feminine corrective balloons and becomes the large black eye of death and, reaching a glittering black arm up through the cracks in the earth, begins to abduct her initiates by the thousands, by the millions.

When we have said too many times *"I'll sleep when I'm dead"*:

The black fish says, *"As you wish."*

~

And so it seemed to me that some kind of feminine reclamation project was clearly in order.

Cutting off the feminine disfigures us all, men and women alike, and fuels toxic masculinity in us all, men and women alike.

And this kind of excavation sounded like just the sort of nice, clean, neutral project we could all get on board with, men and women and nonbinary folks alike—and we wouldn't even have to revisit gender, not really, because it's ultimately about the feminine in *society*, and that's something we can all work on equally, to bring her back into the pantheon of our values, ruling benevolently alongside the masculine. If we are just conscious enough, willful enough, awake enough, and righteous enough, we could all look past our conditioning and work on this problem together, equally, because we are all equal, and Equal means the Same.

There is just one sticky wicket.

Men and women are *not* the same.

Men and women have different brains.
Men and women have different hormones.
Men and women have different immune systems.
Not wildly different, but different enough.

And while it has become impolitic to say so:

Women's bodies—and certain male bodies—are a little bit more *feminine* than most men's.

Something that is obvious to many, and hugely, hugely offensive to others.

And if it didn't matter, reader, you can bet I would not be risking feminist excommunication by picking up this live wire.

But it does matter.

The location of the feminine in the female body, and in certain male bodies, has everything to do with why this problem is not going to solve itself in one happy coed party that we all work on, equally, together, as one. And it has everything to do with why this problem hasn't been solved already.

Despite how unpopular this idea has become, the reality is that hundreds of studies on sex difference support the simple idea that a majority (not all, just a majority) of people born into female bodies have slightly different brain structures, immune systems, and endocrine responses that do seem to explain a slightly (just slightly!) more feminine way of showing up in the world, and instinct for things like connection over domination, empathy over trying to immediately fix a problem, and sensitivity to poor environments instead of a stoic response to poor environments.

In fact, if we're talking womb/tomb, transformation, root systems, the Mother, the underworld, the place of cyclic but ultimately healthy difficulty, nothing is a clearer representative of all this than the female body itself.

We are the world's chrysalis, and the world's most professional cyclists.

As one functional medicine expert in nutrition and hormonal health, Alisa Vitti, explains in her work: a woman's menstrual cycle actually has four distinct phases, which can be interpreted as spring, summer, autumn, and winter. In our follicular and ovulatory weeks—due to the changing concentrations of hormones—we have a bit more energy and a higher libido. And then in our luteal and menstrual weeks—specifically because of those subtle, changing hormones—we are a bit more sensitive and introspective.

You have, I am certain, noticed this.

But normally, as you have also noticed, those second two weeks are not viewed with any kind of admiration or generosity. Women are considered (and consider themselves) bitchy and oversensitive before their period, and then when it finally comes, it's famously considered a Curse. But of course this is entirely a matter of characterization. Through a feminine-positive and underworld-friendly lens, this sensitivity could simply be considered a normal, cyclic opportunity to introspect, to take stock of our lives, to see what's not working, to see what needs to be let go, and to see what needs to be strengthened in the next cycle. We're just never taught to look at it that way.

And while I know this may all sound a bit woo to you, even the least woo among us are aware (along with our boyfriends, partners, and husbands, who are very aware) that we women are not the same all month long. We are generally a bit less tolerant of bullshit the closer we get to our period—even the most stoic, armored women—and we all change rather predictably over the course of the month.

In other words, nearly every single woman for thirty years of her life has an ongoing, lived experience of fourteen days of Upperworld Persephone, and fourteen days of Underworld Persephone.

Thanks to our hormones, we gently wax and wane, every single month, exactly like the moon, exactly like the Earth itself. A healthy relationship with darkness runs right through our reproductive system.

And that should not be a problem at all.

That should not raise your hackles at all.

Cycling is natural and normal and part of life here on planet Earth.

When we cycle well in our lives, flowing between on and off, between going in and going out, between experiencing the light and experiencing the dark, we are healthy. When we cycle, metaphorically speaking, the crops flourish. A person has to pass into the shadowland—in life, frequently—in order to continually dissolve what needs to be dissolved, to retrieve what needs to be retrieved, and to strengthen what needs to be strengthened.

That women cycle should be considered a *strength*.

Connection over domination, empathy over trying to immediately fix a problem, and sensitivity to poor environments instead of a stoic response to poor environments:

These are, at the right times, incredible powers.

And at least for me, when I started reconsidering and rebuilding my esteem for the feminine, the clearer it became that locating "second-class" social values in women's physical bodies was a vile, but extremely effective form of control. There isn't anything a woman can do about it. She's just automatically second-class, unless she hides and disowns and demonizes herself.

Which is precisely what women have done.

As we have gained more and more power, women have more and more made the case that if we are tough enough, armored enough, dispassionate enough, and wear enough pantsuits, then the path to true parity and equal status will open up.

But that isn't what has happened at all.

This posturing has simply caused us to attack ourselves, to demonize our own natural menstrual cycles, and to pooh-pooh our own natural tears, to sniff at the idea that maybe we really are, on the whole, a little bit more collaborative.

When, in fact, we might very well be better served by making the *case* for our powers, without apology.

We might be better served by making the case for sensitivity, and the need to be sensate to a poor environment before things get out of control.

We might be better served by making the case for empathy in our executives, and the need for emotional fluency and healthy emotional expression at the highest levels in order to remain both powerful and benevolent.

Because the alternative is this: if women and femmes and sensitive men won't accept, and own, and be proud of those slight differences, if we are going to treat those differences as verboten, regressive, backwater, and outdated—and yet those differences are real and really do shape some of our behavior, no matter how small:

We are always going to appear broken.

We are always going to be considered, perhaps not overtly, but in the back of everyone's minds, as defective men.

See: Aristotle. See: Freud.

Every time our bodies have a different reaction than men's, especially if it is a more feminine reaction, it will be seen as lesser.

Every time we have a good idea, one that our male and masculine friends genuinely are not having, and that thought is more feminine, it will be seen as soft and unserious.

Every time we react with feeling, in ways that are different from those of even our most emotionally expressive male friends, we will be considered, you guessed it:

Hysterical.

Which—you can't make this stuff up—derives from the Latin word for womb.

Because even though it is invisible, maleness is the standard.

Even though it is invisible, masculine values are the standard.

Even though no doctor will ever mention this to you, the vast majority of clinical trials are still done on white, middle-aged men—in part because the men who design the studies have said that women's menstrual cycles introduce an "X factor" that they feel muddles up the studies.

If Equal means Exactly Like a Man: ladies and some gentlemen, we are quite frankly doomed.

And so as we consider what must be done, I submit to you this:

The fight here is not gender-neutral.

While we do need men and more masculine people to advocate for women and more feminine people, to stick up for us, to make the case for us—we have to be clear-eyed about the fact that they are not going to do this on their own. This problem does not directly affect them, questioning this problem threatens a power structure that directly benefits them, and, have we mentioned, these people are not exactly famous for their great powers of empathy—that is, going down into the dark and experiencing a feeling that is not their own.

We are the ones who are already down here.

We are the ones who know what is going on.

And we need to bring this information back up and into the light.

Loudly, without apology, and probably with some well-earned feminine rage.

If we are smart, instead of disowning our bodies, disowning our femininity, disowning the very things that make us special and valuable—the very aspects that are being so mistreated in medicine and in the workplace, and making us so sick—*this* is the area where we need to lean in.

Into our difference.
Into what is dissimilar, but powerful about us.
Into what we need, which a male may not need.
Into how we present in the world, which is not the same as how a man presents.

We should not do it alone, but we also must not wait for men to do this for us.

It may not sound fair, but dears, if we are waiting for a prince to come down and save us:

That's not how this story goes, and we are going to be waiting forever.

~

I spent months working this out in my mind—alone, bedridden, but mentally (in fits and spurts) quite alive.

My body couldn't move, but I was *deep* in the Nancy Drew phase again, searching, and uncovering, and staking out this new, exciting area of thought. I found all kinds of other women online talking about the same ideas, which was relieving, affirming, and strengthening.

And as I lay in my bed, it was becoming clear to me that the future of medicine was not going to be just 3-D printers and genomics and telemedicine. The other half—the missing half, the "softer" half—that is, an interest in the root causes of illness, in nutrition, in the Mother/microbiome, in self-care, in sleep, in stress, in a more compassionate system—was clearly necessary as well, clearly in demand, and clearly on the rise. Not as a replacement for what we have, but as a coequal partner.

And despite all the expected and inevitable pushback, from all the usual Skeptical suspects (the same skeptics, it should be noted, that have never believed in these illnesses to begin with)—this partnered future actually seemed overwhelmingly logical.

It seemed like this *had* to be the way, or the whole system would topple over. Which indeed can be seen today, as insurance companies buckle under the weight of unprecedented levels of chronic illness, as families buckle under the weight of medical bills, and as the economy groans while trying to support a health care system that in many ways encourages us to stay sick. To continue to exclude diet, the microbiome, lifestyle, and the patient-doctor relationship from our understanding of both the creation of health and the development of disease just does not work, and that isn't some leftist, tree-hugging idea. To exclude food, the microbiome, sleep, and stress from medicine is hugely expensive and fiscally irresponsible to an almost unimaginable degree, for the patient, for the insurance companies, and for the government.

It is illogical, it is inefficient, and it is harmful.

Because we are long overdue for a better, more balanced model.

The Feminine, I think I can say with some certainty, is the missing medicine in Medicine.

And things really seemed to be coming full circle, because I didn't have to think very hard about what that more balanced, partnered, coequal model of health care—one that is interested in the microbiome, the diet, and the root causes of chronic illness—might be.

I already knew it very well, and so do you.

But I'll give you a hint anyway:

It starts with an *f,* and ends with *unctional medicine.*

22

If I had been stuck in the woods with flint and a damp match that kept going out—now, finally, finally, finally, there was a lamp in my hand, held high overhead, and it was burning bright.

I no longer felt like a madwoman waving my arms in the wilderness, shouting about something I had read one time on Yahoo! News. I had found a deep bench of thinkers, doctors, practitioners, and philosophers who were all talking about what I had been trying to understand for so long—and now, in some critical ways, I felt like I was finally standing on solid ground. Solid research ground, solid psychological ground, and solid story ground. Maybe it sounds trite, but understanding really is the first step in any kind of healing—emotional, physical, or otherwise.

And so all this was very nice. Very nice indeed.

But then, of course.

As always, as ever.

Like always, there was one rather large Snag.

The same snag as ever.

This body.

My body.

My poor old body.

Because in reality, my actual life had not evolved at the same pace as my intellectual life.

These halls and caverns I had carved and lit in my mind, this new world of understanding, this huge library of articles and books and archived conversations I had consumed over the course of thirteen months trapped in my bed: it only existed in my head. My understanding and sense of meaning were entirely cerebral, and entirely self-contained. No one around me—literally no one, except perhaps my mother—shared any of these views. Not my friends, not my family, and certainly not my doctors. No one knew what functional medicine was (and if they did, they thought it was nonsense), no one had heard of the HPA axis or microglia, no one wanted to hear a long dialectic on the heroine's journey, and no one wanted to talk about feminine and masculine energies as if that somehow had any bearing on my very serious illness. Everyone, quite naturally, still wanted me to keep questing, to keep fighting, and to keep aiming, firing, and shooting—hoping one day to hit the bullseye.

And so despite all my big ideas about the changes coming in medicine, and the glorious revival of the feminine—in my real, lived life, I was still being shuttled from doctor to doctor, burning hot vaginal exam to burning hot vaginal exam, scalpel to scalpel, surgeon to surgeon. Even though I'd had so, so very many epiphanies up in my good little mind—feminine epiphanies, neuroendocrine-immunological epiphanies, myth-piphanies—I was still a girl in a wheelchair, unable to hold a conversation for very long, unable to make my own food—let alone able to take some grand stand for my vision of the future of medicine. I was weak, in the most literal sense. And like most seriously ill people, I was largely at the mercy of my caretakers and my physicians.

And I must admit, a small, holdout part of me still wanted to see if there was anything—anything at all—that traditional medicine could do for me. I didn't want to be that recalcitrant antimedicine ideologue who stays sick for no reason. And in my ever-trusting heart, I think I believed that because my ideas were becoming less and less radical as they spilled into the mainstream, my physicians would follow suit and have no choice but to open their hearts and minds to a civil, progressive, feminine conversation about my mystery illness.

Why I believed that, I will never know.

~

After a year in bed, I was scooped into a wheelchair and, with my cat in a carrier on my lap, wheeled solemnly through the Tucson airport. From there, I was flown to Washington, D.C., and reinstalled in my childhood bedroom. From there, I was scheduled to see a long laundry list of new specialists. My family and friends were insisting I do this, and so I did.

First, there was a new urogynecologic surgeon, Dr. GYN, a very confident, friendly, thoughtful physician. She was a friend of the family and was seeing me as a favor—and her analysis was helpful. She reviewed the case and hypothesized that perhaps the original assailant, Dr. Damaskus, had done some real damage in my vagina, despite never admitting to any wrongdoing.

Dr. GYN explained that the pelvic area is so delicate and so intricate, some injuries can be extremely difficult to see on a scan— and while she wasn't really sure about it, I liked this explanation, because it was my own pelvic hypothesis, which I had often brought up with my doctors, only to be waved away. I had frequently posited that it felt like there was an actual, mechanical problem in my vagina, on the left side. And that the pain was spreading out from that locus. That is what I had been saying for some time, and I had taken those original sonograms with the slight abnormalities to all those pelvic-pain specialists along the way. And all those pelvic-pain specialists had told me it was nothing, a blip, and not to worry my pretty little vagina.

So I was glad that Dr. GYN was at least open to being on Team Injury.

Sadly, she also said that this potential diagnosis was neither fixable nor confirmable, because beyond repeating those tests, which she felt were unnecessary (they probably wouldn't show anything), there would be nothing left to do about that kind of damage.

But at least we were talking about a real mechanical problem, not just a problem of "perceived" pain. This made it seem like things were going in the right direction and that we were getting down to the root causes.

You know how I feel about root causes.

~

Her next hypothesis, based on hearing from my mother about my long experience with infection and so many other symptoms that indicated an infection of some kind, was that I might have some localized pocket of infection in the pelvis. To test this idea, we could do tiny biopsies of my vagina and of my colon, which would then be sent to the CDC—and while that was a scary prospect, it was also true that I had had a lot of infectious/inflammatory symptoms, and I wanted to solve the mystery as much as anyone else. I agreed to the biopsies—as long as I was put under general anesthesia. No more cutting into my vagina while I was wide awake, thank you.

So about two weeks later, I was all prepped for the surgery in my gown and my hairnet and my hospital booties, with an IV installed in my arm—when the colorectal surgeon, who had been brought on to the case that same day, came bursting into my curtained waiting area.

"Okay, what's going on here?" she said, flipping through my chart.

I looked at her, unsure of how to answer that question.

"I got a call from Dr. GYN and she said she needs me for a biopsy?" she said, looking from me to my mother. "So what's up? Why are we doing this? What are we dealing with here?" she asked, rapid-fire.

I was quite literally minutes away from going under the knife with this woman—and I was so surprised that I had no idea how to respond. There are many reasons we give illnesses names, but this is one of them. One should really be able to answer the simple question: What's wrong? But I couldn't, and I started stammering about its being a complicated case, which no one had been able to figure out, but some people thought I might have an infection, and I also had chronic fatigue syndrome, and CRPS, and maybe fibromyalgia, but I also had really bad pelvic pain, which had all started with an injury, and—

"Jesus Christ," she said, exasperated, and swooped back out.

My mother went out to speak with her, and this seemed to bother the doctor even more. She did not like being called in to pinch-hit for another surgeon when she had never seen the patient personally and really didn't know what was going on. And as I sat there in my booties listening to my mother try to explain my impossible case, and listening to the surgeon huff and puff and express her extreme displeasure at being involved with so little preparation, my heart started to pound in my chest. *Don't cry, don't cry, don't cry*, I thought. *It's going to be fine. Everything is fine. You just have to trust. Trust the Universe!* I focused on trusting the Universe.

Suddenly, Dr. GYN herself swooped in, a ball of energy.

"Ready? Let's do this!" she exclaimed.

I looked at her with alarm, and tried to explain that the other surgeon seemed to be confused, and she said, "Oh, don't worry, I'll walk her through the whole thing. You're going to be just fine. You've got me!"

Surely the most cheerful urogynecologic surgeon in existence.

"Are you sure?" I asked, looking tragic.

"Of course I'm sure. I'm very good at my job, Ms. Sarah. Relax and it will be over before you know it."

She smiled, and I felt a small bit better.

And then, given the green light, the nurses bustled in, helped heave me up onto the gurney, and before I knew it, the black anesthesia mask was descending onto my face and I was counting backward from ten, floating off into a sea of propofol.

And when I woke up, I was in so much pain and shaking so hard, I bit straight through my tongue.

~

When I came out of anesthesia, there was an expected stinging sensation in my vagina, but—and I regret to tell you this—it was my poor little anus that inexplicably felt to be on fire. I lifted up the hospital blanket and saw that I was bleeding onto the table. I was given pain medication and helped into an adult diaper. And as the diaper pulled at my skin, I felt searing pain—in my anus. Which did not make any sense, and I asked a nurse why my anus hurt so much. And she said:

"Because they biopsied your anus!"

Like a deer's anus caught in the headlights, I stared back at her, aghast.

Because they weren't supposed to biopsy my anus.
They were supposed to biopsy my colon.
Nobody said anything about biopsying my anus.

And this discrepancy might seem trivial to those without quite so many colorectal problems in their lives, so let me clarify. You can't actually feel a biopsy of your colon once it's over—the colon is not innervated with the same kind of sensory nerves as our skin and extremities—and this is why a biopsy of the colon is generally not a big deal, indeed the reason I had agreed to it.

Your anus, on the other hand, you can very much feel.

Furthermore, *if you have CRPS in your anal nerves*—literally the world's most severe chronic pain syndrome—*and also have to use said CRPS anus twenty times a day because of your severe bowel disorder*—then cutting a one-by-two-centimeter divot in such an anus—without talking it over with the patient—is in no uncertain terms a monumental mistake.

This accidental wound took about six weeks to stop feeling like I was shitting boric acid and cayenne pepper twenty-six times a day. Every single time I sat on the toilet, I literally screamed in pain. I had to wear a diaper with an ice pack inside it. They gave me painkillers—which, as always, caused my muscles to ache terribly and made me vomit with some frequency.

And when I expressed my feelings of outrage in my follow-up appointment (is there another emotion when someone cuts into your anus by accident?)—Dr. Anus, as we must now call her, told me to calm down and stop being so emotional.

She gave no apology, and said that she had made a game-time decision to biopsy the anus because she thought it could only be helpful. Dr. GYN had not stopped her. And anyway, if I wanted my case solved, I needed to put on my big-girl panties and do whatever it took.

I would later find out that Dr. Anus is roundly considered by colleagues and patients alike to be a pretty big asshole herself. A bit of a Gregory House, if you will. A good surgeon, but famously uncaring, brusque, and mean.

Regardless, all the biopsies came back negative.

~

Following that incident, I was shuttled between five more doctors, who argued over whether or not I should get an ileostomy (installation of an external poo bag), the one operation at that point that I was actually asking for—begging for—so I could at least stop the insanity of the daily colonoscopy preps/Bowel Olympics.

But then, after eight separate visits, it was decided—solely based on how I had "overreacted" to the accidental anal biopsy—that I was too sensitive and unpredictable to risk it.

One of the colorectal surgeons recommended I try the Mayo Clinic.

And when I told him I'd just come from there, he suggested I try a psychiatrist.

~

Next I was sent down the line to Pain Doctor #1, who was actually a very nice man.

The plan was to experiment with nerve blocks up and down the spine—painful procedures involving long needles inserted into the nerve plexes of the spinal cord while facedown, naked, and awake on the operating table. I had tried these years before, but we decided to try them again. We did these once a week over the course of the summer, and they *did* provide blessed relief, but their numbing effects lasted only about twelve hours each.

In the wake of this failure, Pain Doctor #1 then referred me to Pain Doctor #2, a pelvic-pain specialist, who was not, actually, a very nice man.

He disagreed with Dr. GYN and did not think I had sustained any damage in the initial incident with Dr. Damaskus. He believed that my pain signals had become ingrained in my brain and nervous system, and were not "real" per se. They felt real—he was not denying that—but they were not due to any actual inflammation or damage.

What he recommended for this was a spinal cord stimulator—or a radio implanted in my back next to my spinal cord with up to sixteen long wires threaded subcutaneously over the problem areas. The wires buzz, and this distracts your brain so it doesn't send as many pain signals. This was not a new idea, but it seemed like the time had come to give it a try.

Pain Doctor #2 then sent me back to Pain Doctor #1 to see what he thought about getting a stimulator, and Pain Doctor #1 agreed we should try it. He explained that there was a trial procedure that Pain Doctor #2 would perform first to see if I were a good candidate for the final surgery. And Pain Doctor #1 helpfully described that procedure in detail to me, explaining that it would involve a single trial wire inserted next to my spinal cord, and that wire would attach to an external controller, worn in a fanny pack for a week. That relatively noninvasive procedure with the single wire was called a "percutaneous test."

I agreed to do a percutaneous test.

I arrived at the hospital for the procedure, to be performed by Pain Doctor #2, on September 14, 2014, at 5:00 a.m. My mother, brother, and father were there—all of whom had high hopes that this could really help. They had wanted me to get this kind of machine implanted for a long time. They gave me thumbs-up signs and wished me luck as I drifted off again into that welcome ocean of anesthesia.

When I next opened my eyes, groggy and confused, I could see the outlines of my parents, I could see what looked like Pain Doctor #2, and I could see the nurse, the fluorescent lights, the beige walls, and the IV going into my arm.

But most important, for the first time in over a decade—I felt no pain.

Pain Doctor #2 smiled with satisfaction as he asked me a list of questions regarding my pain levels. Zero, zero, zero! I said, heart singing. I could not believe it, and I slurred my undying gratitude and thanks to him for saving me.

And then, the anesthesia started to wear off.

As my senses started to stir and come alive again, one nerve after another started firing, and my brain started to process that something was actually quite wrong.

At first, I thought I must be confused—I have an oversensitive brain, after all, and I was also quite loopy. But as I tried to move, my sensations were unmistakable. It felt like everything—my vagina, my pelvic floor, and both buttocks—was burning up. I tried to sit up but was stunned by an electric network of pain zigzagging through my whole lower half. The room spun, but there was no mistaking—the vagina, the pelvic floor, and both buttocks felt like they had somehow been sliced open and then glued back together.

And as it turned out, they had.

In the next few minutes, I learned that while I was under general anesthesia, Pain Doctor #2 had performed a *totally different surgery* than the one Pain Doctor #1 had described. Instead of a single wire alongside the spine, my pelvis was now filled with a warren of wires. Pain Doctor #2 had drilled long tines up through the pelvic floor (the CRPS pelvic floor), alongside both sides of the vagina (the CRPS vagina), driving both wires through the pelvic bowl all the way to the top of my left buttock (the CRPS left buttock). There, he bisected that (CRPS) cheek with a large incision to bury a packet of radio wires. Then he tunneled some of those wires under the skin across the left-side (CRPS) buttock, the (CRPS) sacrum, and all the way over to the right-side (CRPS) buttock, where two large cables punctured the (CRPS) skin, exited, and were connected to an external controller, worn in a fanny pack.

The fanny pack was the only part of the procedure that even remotely resembled the surgery I had agreed to.

And when I burst into tears at this news, Pain Doctor #2 immediately prescribed a powerful opioid and I drifted back off to sleep.

He explained to my parents that I simply needed to get some rest, get used to the device, and soon I would be experiencing the benefits.

The next day, when I called Pain Doctor #1 to get some explanation for what in the actual fuck was going on, he asked me to describe the incisions, which I did, at which point he just started saying over and over again, "Oh no, oh no, oh no."

And so I learned that Pain Doctors #1 and #2 had not communicated properly. Much like Dr. GYN and Dr. Anus had not communicated properly. Pain Doctor #2 had performed an outdated procedure called a "staged trial"—something tantamount to doing the entire surgery, where you put *all* the wires in, not just a test wire—a step you only, only, only take if you feel certain the device will work.

And why anyone would feel certain of anything in my particular case, I do not know.

But he had. And he thought Pain Doctor #1 had described that surgery to me, and that I knew what I was getting into.

And practically speaking, there was nothing we could do about it now. The thing was in.

He told me that ripping the apparatus out would just cause more pain, and advised me to keep it in to see if I got any relief at all. So I did.

And in the long course of my historically painful illness, I have never been in so much pain in all my life.

~

So, reader.

I admit I feel a little bad for you.

Because who in the whole wide world wants to hear *More Colo-Vago-Uro Scary Stories to Tell in the Dark?*

Not you, I suspect.
And not me, I know.

So here is where I'd like to take the needle off the record.

Enough.

Enough.
Enough.
Enough.

We have all had enough.

I hope you are tired of hearing these violating, nauseating, nightmare stories, over and over again.

I certainly am, and I am also tired of having to tell them.
And tired of having to live them.
And tired of having to relive them.

And so, I come to you with good news.

This is the last time I am ever going to tell you a story like this.

We will put aside the rant about medical mistakes being extremely common (the third leading cause of death in the United States, just behind heart disease and cancer) and we will put aside the rant about pelvic pain being routinely mishandled, and discounted, in the most egregious ways (if you are a pelvic-pain patient reading this, you know this too well), and we will even put aside the fact that "Oh no, oh no, oh no" is just about the last phrase you want to hear any surgeon say, ever.

We can put all of that aside for now, because in the end, this incident turned out to be one of the most important things that has ever happened to me.

It turned out that I needed a Last Straw, and a True Rock Bottom.
And drilling long wires into my vagina without my permission turned out to be my own personal last straw, and the bottomest of rock bottoms.

This time when I was carried back to my bed to recuperate from yet another botched procedure—shaking, lips chapped, lying on my side to avoid all the wounds, clawing at my pillow because of the extraordinary pain, crying so hard no sound came out—this time instead of my hope light going out, or despair taking over, or my spirit leaving my body and floating out the window—this time, it was as if a small force field started to emanate from within me, and around me—a glistening, titanium shield—a near-mystical force that seemed to be coming from that deep and healthy place within me, a wellspring that had made itself known a few memorable, almost magical times in my long illness.

It was that deep and healthy place of *fuck you.*
The divine messenger of appropriate anger.

My friend.
My ally.
My protector.
From whom I had somehow grown apart.
Again.

But now, I was shimmering, crackling with rage.

I felt profoundly violated, as I believe anyone who goes to sleep and wakes up with surprise wires drilled into their vagina would feel.

I felt furious, and simultaneously afraid in a deep, reptilian way.

How could this be happening?

Again?

Was there no way to be treated properly in the medical system, if you also happened to have the overlay of this kind of mysterious disease?

Was there a magnet inside of me that removed the word *no* from the physician's credo "Do no harm"?

Naturally, Caroline Myss floated into my mind for a moment to explain to me, again, that I was simply a bad person, addicted to suffering, attracting tragedies because bad luck is drawn in by bad energy, and I obviously had bad energy, bad ju-ju, bad vibes, bad karma. But this time, as Caroline drifted toward me with those outstretched, insidious New Age thoughts—to my surprise, my fuck you titanium shield bounced her right off, and she ricocheted clear across the Maryland sky.

For a moment, I longed to be back with my books, hidden away with Clarissa Pinkola Estés and Marion Woodman, wondering why I couldn't escape to some female colony where ample-bodied women hold and take care of one another and don't think surgery and medication are the only options. Why couldn't I just find some soft place to live where I would be accepted as a person deserving of care, where I could at least get the palliative treatment I needed? We do that for so many diseases, why not this one? Why does it have to be this way? Why don't things ever, ever change?

And as all these feelings pulsed, shaking the windows and rattling the walls, I allowed myself to feel them all. The rage, the grief, the anger, the sadness, the fear. I allowed myself to feel fury—storming, destructive, ugly fury. I allowed myself to feel the terror of a victim—weak, trembling, self-pitying, vulnerable terror. And I allowed myself to feel grief—a profound sadness for my tiny, precious flame of hope that a thousand people in white coats seemed so intent on blowing out, again and again and again. These emotions spilling, pouring, and churning out of me were so ferocious, I felt I could make the sky darken, the clouds roil, and lightning to crackle and shoot from every nerve, every vein, every wound.

And all I could think was:

A rape.
   A trauma.
      An illness.
         A death.

Loss, search, return.
Descent, mystery, ascent.
Destruction, gathering, rebirth.

Everything I had been reading about and beginning to under-stand—it was playing out in real time all around me, again. A mon-strously masculine system for a profoundly feminine problem. Knives, scalpels, pills, sterility, and institutional detachment from feeling—for a problem of vaginas, hormones, feces, trauma, and a kind of pain and sensitivity that absolutely, absolutely, absolutely requires empa-thy, patience, nourishment, listening, and care.

And even though I knew all that in my mind, there I was, stuck in the same situation—again. I was *still* waiting to be saved. Or waiting for someone else to swoop in and save me from the scalpel wielders. Or waiting for my family to suddenly realize that their way of doing medicine wasn't right for people like me. Or waiting for one of my doctors to say, "Wait a minute! What about the one neuroendocrine-immunological ring to rule them all? Great Scott, we're doing this *all wrong!*"

It was like I had been sold into marriage with traditional medi-cine, and we all believed there was nothing I could do about it, and it was ultimately for the best. And I needed to keep going back again and again, even if he was violent, even if he said I was to blame. Because owing to the tremendous respect and authority accorded to him and his stature, he could get away with terrible behavior. Again and again and again. And it was explained away—*he means well; this is just the way things are; you're lucky to have him at all*—again and again and again.

And, just as in the case of being married against your will—or, for that matter, in the case of any injustice—*What you resist, persists* is in fact atrocious advice.

New Age, positive-thinking hero Eckhart Tolle's admonition that "the only appropriate responses to life are acceptance, enjoyment, and enthusiasm" is just categorically, laughably, tragically untrue.

My problem was that the medical system really and truly was not set up for illnesses like mine, which intentionally or not, resulted in extremely bad—and often explicitly abusive—medical care.

That was a fact. People might not like that fact, they might be confronted and offended by that fact, but it was still a fact.

Everyone with ME/CFS, complex regional pain syndrome, sick building syndrome, post-treatment Lyme disease syndrome, and all the rest knows that this is a fact.

And so my biggest problem wasn't that I couldn't think enough positive thoughts, or find enough silver linings, or grasp that the night is often darkest before the dawn.

My problem was that I was all nonviolence and no resistance.

I was suffering acutely from the Curse of the Good Girl.

The accommodater. The pleaser. The bender. The achiever. The gold star winner.

That deep but blocked place of *fuck you*, in my case, was a source of profound health.
It was the good kind of anger.
The good kind of boundary.
The fire that helps you protect yourself, stand up for yourself, and advocate for yourself.

And if you don't have this, in a system that is not set up for you:

Dear, you are completely screwed.

A "profound lack of anger" is no gold-star achievement.

In fact, it occurred to me as a thousand lightning bolts flew around the room and the wind howled and the rain went sideways: my profound lack of anger was profoundly damaging me.

I had always been the Good Girl, and it had served me well enough for the twenty years before I got sick. Because people like being pleased, people like being accommodated, and people like you to stay positive. They reward you for it. Being Good is a way of staying likable in order to get by. But when I got sick and was told incorrectly that my illness was actually a hallucination, or a personality disorder—well, I was now in a bit of a bind. I was being a good girl, but it didn't matter. They still were saying terrible, untrue things about me, no matter how good I was. And yet, if I was angry about this wrongful treatment, and especially if I made a fuss about it—I would just prove everyone right and prove I had some kind of emotional problem. Anyone without power knows this double bind too well. And I did what we all tend to do—I went out of my way to bend over backward, being kind, generous, pleasing, intelligent, compliant, and obedient with all of my doctors. I genuinely thought that this would help me. I thought if they just saw that I was a nice, normal young lady, they would stop treating me like a snaggletoothed, sniveling, clutching, parasitic malingerer.

They didn't stop treating me that way, but somehow that didn't change my behavior.

And when I moved into alternative healing, I received that exact same message again and again and again—that if I was angry or resistant to anything at all, then I was creating my own illness and I wasn't a good spiritual seeker. To be angry—at all—was to be the spiritually snaggletoothed, sniveling, clutching, parasitic malingerer.

And so as I lay there in my childhood bed for the thousandth time, shaking, shaking, shaking, and could feel that fury coursing through me—hot and fierce—I was beginning to realize:

It felt *good*.

It was the feeling of being *alive*.
It was the feeling of responding appropriately to life.

This time, lying in my bed in the same situation I had been in so many times, something was different from all the times before.

This time, I knew better.

This time, my lamp was on, and I wasn't lost.

And while I might still be weak in my body, something had happened in those twenty-four months of reading books with stories that actually reflected something true, and deep, and old back to me in the mirror.

I had slowly stopped rejecting myself.
I had slowly stopped divorcing myself.
I had slowly stopped bending and folding and shaming and contorting.

And now, though it took a violent nudge to fully realize it, it was clear that it was my duty, and my duty alone, to protect this union between me and me at all costs.

I did have a weakness, and it was running the show.

My weakness was that I was being too fucking nice.

And I was mistaken in believing it would get me anywhere but the exact same place I had been before.

I was constantly trying to see the good in my doctors—to look for their best intentions, to honor the incredible difficulty of their job, to respect their flawed humanity, which is the same as my own flawed humanity, and to appreciate their incredible breadth of knowledge, skill, and training, for which I really *do* have such tremendous respect. But in the process, I was completely discounting my own importance, my own difficult job, and my own breadth of knowledge. I was discounting that I really might know more about myself and my body than they did. That I might actually know what was best for me, and that there really was something profoundly wrong with the medical system, at least in relationship to cases like mine. I wasn't wrong about that. And to declare it wasn't arrogance or meanness or violence or being a spoiled brat—it was just the truth. There was a real problem, and it was really hurting me, and I deserved to be protected instead of carved up again and again, "for my own good."

Not standing up for myself—honestly, not even realizing that this was a situation where I could or should stand up for myself—was keeping me locked, permanently, in hell.

I thought of my father, and that even though he was the one pushing me for more surgery, more doctors, more intervention, if the tables were turned and he had been treated this way, cut, sliced, shamed, and ignored, he would have stood up a long time ago and told everyone to go fuck themselves.

And I thought of my mother, who felt torn between keeping me in the system and experimenting outside the system with alternative therapies—and I thought about how the tables actually *had* been turned for her (my mother had a period of WOMIdom back in the day—which was discounted for five years by her colleagues before she got appropriate care)—and that she, too, had fought for herself, and fought to find the right medical team, the right kinds of doctors, until she finally got treated in the right ways.

And I realized that even though my parents were pretty good at standing up for themselves, they didn't want their darling daughter to do it. They wanted her to submit. They wanted her to do what she was told. They wanted her to be saved.

And of course, reader, this is not a new story.

But lying there with my vagina sliced open, and my wires dangling, and my incisions burning, and my fanny pack chafing, one thing finally seemed abundantly clear.

No one was going to save this darling daughter but me.

There would be no march, no ribbon, no book, no Dumbledore, no Hagrid—no parents, no heroic friends, and no epic romantic life-saving cliffhanger.

I needed to save myself.

I needed to be Hagrid, Dumbledore, parent, friend, and epic romance. I needed to burst through the door and send the Dursleys tumbling in the corner. I needed to be the one throwing a protective shield around myself, and standing up to the people who did not know what they were doing, did not have any training for what to do about patients like myself, and were hurting me, over and over and over again. I needed to grow myself ten feet tall, and I needed to announce to the Muggles that I did not belong under the staircase—and was, in fact, the girl who lived.

I knew that, but as you may know, the gulf between Knowing and Doing is deep and wide.

Lying in bed with my eyes pressed shut, that story that had been knocking, and then banging, and then hammering at my door my entire life—a story I had only just started to understand, in my mind, book by book, article by article, conversation by conversation—that story was now sending a huge, flaming, boar-headed battering ram to the gates, with one loud and now finally clear message.

Open. The fucking. Gate.

It was time to let the feminine story of dying into life come through—and to come through *me*.

The story of initiation into the earth, into the feminine, into the cycler, the ecologist, the descender, the excavator, the reweaver, the nourisher, the healer—the seat of life, who is *also* the Gorgon, the ugly one, the monster, and the one who kills all the crops just to get her daughter back. Isis, Inanna, Demeter, Persephone, La Loba—sometimes life-giving, kind, springlike, and beautiful—and sometimes hideous, ferocious, resistant, and unliked.

It was time for me, as Virginia Woolf would say, to kill the angel in the house.

To let the underworld story come through, now, down in my body—nurturer, nourisher, caregiver, Gorgon-composting-feces-monster and all.

Out of my mind, where it was safe, and down into my real, lived life.

And even though things seemed so bad there in my bed, so destroyed, and so hopeless, I knew deep down in my undead bones that I had already been through the Loss—again and again and again—and I also knew that I had been through the Search—for years and years and years—and now, as the floor rumbled and the lights blinked and the smoke rose, curling off my skin, it was clear to me that the next phase was now, finally at hand.

I opened my eyes with stone-cold clarity and thought:

It is time to get the hell out of Hell.

III

23

Dear reader, I promised you an end to the sad stories, and I am a woman of my word.

So before we say anything else, I want to fast-forward and stop four years after Dr. Oops drilled the wrong wires into my pelvis, five years after Dr. Jekyll became Mr. Hyde between two stirrups, and almost six years after the Great Crash and the pools of saliva on the bathroom floor.

Fast-forward to right now.

Right now, as I tap away at the keyboard, I am not dictating from within a body collapsed on itself.
Right now, I am not shaved, shorn, and tucked into bed.
Right now, I am not wearing a muumuu with golden retrievers on it.

Right now, I am sitting up.
Right now, I am *writing at a desk.*

It is a beautiful, sunny day in Arizona, the creosote and the desert sage are perfuming the air after last night's monsoon, and Mathilde is curled at my feet in a hexagon of light.
This morning, I woke early and did some simple yoga outside.
Last night, I ate a meal of real, solid food.
Last weekend, I walked around a museum, sat in a café, and drank tea.
In a few weeks, I am scheduled to play my third Wolf Larsen show this year.

And a few weeks after that, I will sit around a Thanksgiving table with my friends and my family—my third holiday spent upright, among other human beings.

No wheelchairs.
No round-the-clock nursing.
No bleak, blank stare out the window.

Am I all the way better?
Oh Hades, no.

But I am not dead.
I am not even undead.

I am alive.

And so, if up until this very moment I have been telling you the rip-roaring mystery-whodunit of how I got to be dead (or undead)—now I'd like to complete the myth and unspool the mystery-whodunit of how someone like me comes back to life.

Because after all this time, I have finally come to realize:

A near-supernatural ability to rise up from the dead—
That is, and has always been, my real superpower.

And my dear reader:
It's probably yours, too.

~

Before we proceed, I am going to have to ask you to gird your loins. In order to tell you the story of how someone like me comes back to life, we have to strike into some semiprescriptive territory—a very fraught and uncertain part of the mystery illness story. So before we dive in, we also have to lay out a few qualifications, caveats, warnings, cautions, stipulations, and provisos.

Because prescriptive territory is tricky terrain. Cynics to the right of us—*there's nothing you can do; the health movement is bullshit; take your meds and shut the fuck up*—idealists to the left—*you can do anything you set your mind and your mini trampoline to!*—and a personal library piled high in my home, bursting with advice—reams, stacks, towers of advice. Indeed, I imagined this very moment for years and years—a decade spent dreaming about the sunny day I would finally stand on the mountaintop and deliver the Perfect Plan, the WOMI Way, the Ramey Method, calling out, "Follow me, friends, for I know the good word!" I have imagined you, the reader, in my mind's eye—the mysteriously ill, my comrade, my secret twin—and also the brothers, and cousins, and fathers, and other friends-of-WOMIs (FWOMIs) who might be reading—imagining just what it is that you need to hear, just what it is you need to know, and just what words would be the most exact, most right, most soothing, and most comforting balm.

Because I want to help you.
I want to heal you.
Dang it all—*I want to save you.*

I'm afraid for some of us, that impulse never goes away.

But of course, I can't. Every time anyone thinks they've got the mystery illness map moderately well plotted, it shifts. Every time I think I couldn't read another book about health, or the future of health, or people like us, a new study comes out, a new book hits the bestseller list, or a new myth-busting article about the microbiome starts trending, and my view expands or contracts. And every time I think I know something for sure, I also know for sure that someone is about to shake the health landscape out like a quilt, slightly rearranging the mountains, fields, and the forests.

This is the nature of a complex problem.
Indeed, isn't it the nature of science?

It's supposed to evolve, it is never exact, and the entire premise of the scientific enterprise is iterative—always expanding, and deepening, and sometimes changing radically. This seems to me a reasonable set of expectations when it comes to working out a complex problem, in that nuances and subtleties and layers and paradoxes should be anticipated—not cause for suspicion or outrage.

Therefore, because the mysterious illnesses are *so* complex—if we are to take on the beginnings of the emerging solutions here at all, we have to agree to hold those solutions loosely.

First of all, as noted, no two WOMIs are the same. Reader, you could be a WOMI 1 or a WOMI 5, which are profoundly different experiences. You could have rheumatoid arthritis, or lupus, or Crohn's, or celiac, or multiple sclerosis, or Hashimoto's, or Raynaud's, or Sjögren's, or Type 2 diabetes—all related, but all quite different. You could have low stomach acid or high stomach acid, PCOS or Ehlers-Danlos, Epstein-Barr or Lyme, mast cell activation syndrome or fibromyalgia. You could have a problem with yeast, or bad bacteria, or parasites, or viruses, or mold. You could have a problem with mercury, or lead, or aluminum, or cadmium, or antimony, or chromium, or iron. You could have a deficiency in vitamin A, or B1, or B2, or B3, or B5, or B6, or B12, or C, or D, or E, or K.

You could have one of these things.
You could have many of these things.
You could have most of these things and more, you unlucky minx.

The WOMI Continuum is real, and we mysteriously ill really do contain multitudes.

In this book, we are not just talking about the narrow definition of ME/CFS—sudden, disabling fatigue usually coming on after a trauma to the system. We're talking about the much larger and much more complex web of problems and symptoms and illnesses and diagnoses that are clearly all connected. Our working theory is one of aggregate stress to the body, resulting in a variety of broken-down barriers, inflammation, and a multitude of disrupted systems—and so right out of the gate we understand that there is an awful lot that can go wrong for this patient. When you have a hyperpermeable intestinal lining and dysfunctional immunity, what can get past a normally well-guarded perimeter is legion, not singular. Likewise, if you have a disrupted endocrine system, a disrupted immune system, a disrupted gastrointestinal system, and a disrupted nervous system—the many ways those systems can go out of balance are legion, not singular. And if this is our working theory, then each WOMI should be *expected* to have a different permutation of the problem—a different endocrine problem, a different immune problem, a different gastrointestinal problem, and a different problem in the nervous system—and that is normal and to be anticipated.

This is, in your narrator's very strong opinion, why we all look somewhat the same, but why we are also all perplexingly unique.

Mystery solved.

Thus, the concept of writing to "you" or "your daughter" doesn't exactly work. We're all so different. Not only is this not a singular illness, with a singular culprit, it is also impossible to know where anyone is on the path—the many-cycled path. Has this been going on for our patient for twenty years, or did she just begin her descent? Has she tried everything from Ayurvedic enemas to special diets to cryogenic ice baths—or has she tried nothing, and remains deeply skeptical of making any changes? Is her cabinet full of tinctures and smudge sticks from deep in the Peruvian rain forest, or is it full of steroids, antidepressants, acid blockers, and Ambien?

Or is she a mix of these two types, vacillating between extreme belief and extreme cynicism?

For all I know, she could be absolutely anywhere on this spectrum, and so writing to you or to her, as if WOMIs were distinct entities, known quantities, with a fixed illness—well, it just doesn't work. Which is the big, inconvenient wrinkle that makes so much of the available health advice—the abundant, overflowing, trumpeting, blinking, blaring, heaping piles of advice on the Internet, in your in-box, in advertisements, in workshops, and in the bookstore—so misleading.

I do not wish to do that to you. I am exhausted by the rancor and the overpromising, and I suspect you may be too.

So instead, we're going to circle back to my central, guiding principle:

The Common Denominator.
The Pattern.
The Big Picture.

I know that taking this 50,000-foot-view approach is a little frustrating because it is necessarily imprecise—but if we zoom in too close, we end up leaving out large sections of the Continuum. I could spend the next fifty pages delving into the complexities of treating Lyme, but where would that leave our friends with endometriosis, irritable bowel syndrome, and Hashimoto's? Or our friends with fibromyalgia and mast cell activation syndrome? Or our very, very best friends, those of you with outrageous cases of vulvodynia?

For me, after I had gotten back to this miraculous place of being able to drive my own car and sit at a desk and sing a few songs for an audience every few months (that is, still pretty disabled by any standard, but achieving monumental wins for the not-walking dead), I spent a long time examining what I had done. Because this time around I had not gotten better because of anything fringe, wild, or extreme. This time, I had focused on the common-denominator behaviors and treatments that had always worked for me in the past, the behaviors and treatments that all the best data points to, and the behaviors and treatments that I had seen work for so many of my healed and partially healed compatriots.

In broad strokes—from mindset, to diet, to medication, to self-care—what I implemented is what almost everyone I know who makes real progress with these illnesses implements. Not only that, but there is a progression in how the whole thing is put together.

There are stages.
Stations, if you will.

Details do matter, and everyone's path will be filled with particulars and idiosyncrasies and things that work or don't work specifically for them. That's important. You get to have your specific thing that works for you, but doesn't work for me, and vice versa. You will have your major internal stressor and I will have mine. But if we can't get the *gist* of the thing down first—if we can't find common ground and a basic, shared path—then the war between the different health-movement factions will go on forever. And all that popular, clickable, polarizing approach does is to jerk everyone back and forth, leaving us all suffering from terrible health-advice whiplash, overwhelmed, growing more and more cynical every day. When the Internet blows these discrepancies between the tribes out of proportion (which it does with a kind of wild, adolescent glee), it just muddles a very important question:

What is a WOMI supposed to *do*?
Right now?
Starting today?

Because she can't just do nothing and expect it to get better.
And she can't just wing it.
And if she does wing it, I can all but guarantee she will either end up on ten medications and just as sick as when she started, or hanging in her garage from a pair of gravity boots, anointed in frankincense, counting mala beads, chanting *I am fabulous*—just as sick as when she started.

It doesn't have to be this way anymore.

Even though there is no 100 percent foolproof, superslick plan where we all get miraculously better, we definitely know enough now to give patients more than Prozac and a raised eyebrow. We know enough now to buffer some of the very worst of the symptoms for many of these patients. It is a work in progress, I am the first to admit. *I* am a work in progress. We all are. Treatment for the mystery illnesses is obviously a work in progress—and no one can or should tell you otherwise. Most of us are either entirely underground or have only one leg and a wing sticking awkwardly out of the chrysalis.

The Return has a slightly imaginary, gossamer quality to it—as if it's being born right now.

But that's just how it is. It *is* being born. Right now.

We can see the shape and the contours of the thing—and for so many of us who have been so lost, so unseen, and so untreated, or maltreated, or half-treated, even one fragile wing waving in the morning light is a real glimmer of hope.

That's what I'm here for.

I am going to take a stand for the common denominator, for the outlines of the emerging map, no matter how homemade and janky it is. As you go along, I hope you will edit and adapt and collaborate with me to make the map work for you, your sister, your coworker, or your daughter. If you agree to stay open to me, I very much agree to stay open to you. In my experience, messy as it is, that is the best way forward.

So with no further ado, let us start at the beginning of the end.

Back inside my titanium shield, a hundred thousand raging emotions coursing through my neuroendocrine-immunological system, Medusa throttles fully engaged.

We begin here, because the first thing to make clear beyond all shadows of all doubts is that my return to the land of the living was not set in motion because of a miracle, or a surgery, or a boyfriend, or a yoga pose, or a cure. Nor was my return to the land of the living because I passively waited and watched and saw. And for *sure* my return to the land of the living was not because I generated enough positive thoughts and the angels finally smiled.

I do not want there to be any mistake about this.

My return, instead, began at the precise moment in time that I unapologetically, unabashedly, and unrelentingly commenced in the full and passionate embrace of some wonderfully negative thoughts.

And so that is where our resurrection story begins.

24

We are back inside the electrical storm.

Windows, broken. Sun, blotted. Caroline Myss, banished.

Me, iridescent with rage.

And inside the typhoon, a real-time, aggressive, and permanent change reticulating in my brain. My neurons were shifting and changing in a moment of acute stress, and indeed it was that healthy and adaptive belief out of which everything else on this map began to flow freely, and that was:

Embrace Hades.

No surprise, I know—however if I, heroine enthusiast, was not actually applying this idea in my own life, your average WOMI probably isn't either. Welcoming the underworld is rare, and it is extremely different from the more typical, heroic health quest she has likely constructed for herself. Installing these new metaphors and symbols and themes—accepting that this dark, feminine story is now unfolding in and around her—this is very difficult. And so it bears repeating:

Embrace Hades.

A wide-ranging, fairly lofty idea to apply to a real, lived life, so let me paint you a picture.

The journey into Hades is the journey inward—into the individual, into her body, into her culture.

The journey into Hades is the journey to the place where darkness not only dominates every scene, but also the place where darkness is taken seriously, and must not be demonized. Illnesses, emotions, symptoms—these become clues in the shadows to be understood as valid and vital guides, giving her information that she must become able to sit with, and slowly decode, and eventually learn from.

The journey into Hades is the journey down, into the root system—where problems are examined at the level of origin, and that knowledge (no matter how inconvenient) is then brought back up to the light of day in order to make the necessary adjustments.

Thus, the journey into Hades is the journey to the place of real transformation—using the information from the underworld to change herself, and help others change—slowly, steadily, surely, cyclically—with one clear and perhaps unexpected goal:

Health.

Hades is about health.

Going down into the root system—physical, emotional, cultural—is about health.

Physical, emotional, cultural.

But make no mistake:

No one likes Hades.
No one likes to compost *themselves*.
No one likes to accept a path that is inherently dark and confusing and confronting, and structured to burn away certain aspects, and beliefs, and behaviors that one may hold very dear, even if they are unhealthy. People do not like human winter. And most people do not want to exact human winter on the people around them—especially in such a sun/smiles/self-reliant/hero-positive culture.

Too bad.

A WOMI *is* on the underground path.
It's just what's happening.

She knows it, I know it.
And she has to accept it.

Because if she is underground and keeps trying to go about life in an aboveground manner, things will just get worse and worse.

If she snuffs out her pain before learning from it, she will never get to the root cause—and if she never gets to the root cause, the problem will generally be destined to repeat.

If she is floating away on a periwinkle cloud of positivity or denial, she is likely to remain deactivated and unable to truly engage with the gnarly and difficult realities of her life.

If she is passively expecting that she is going to be saved by the heroes of the medical establishment, she will be repeatedly horrified to learn that her doctor is, in fact, the March Hare.

If she is anticipating her path is going to be linear and clean, not cyclical and messy—she will feel hopeless and angry every time she is not swiftly and immediately cured.

And for absolute sure: if she doesn't expect to change herself at all, then she is going to stay stuck in the underworld, and the sick root system will continue to hurt her and others like her.

Descent, disintegration, loss, compost, surrender, and death.

Lengthy, patient, and scrappy exploration, excavation, and gathering of knowledge.

Taking action to correct what does not make her stronger, and laying claim to what truly fortifies her—otherwise known as realignment, rooting, nourishment, connection, and growth.

These are the motifs that will repeat for her.
Again and again and again.
And they will scare and disappoint her.
Again and again and again.

Because she is not prepared for this journey.
No one is.

We do not live in a heroine's world.

But what I have observed (again and again and again) in my own life, and in the lives of all WOMIs, MOMIs, and HOMIs who are able to regrow themselves, even a little:

Once you accept that you are down the rabbit hole, and once you accept the heavy burden of having to look at the roots of your own problems—bravely, frequently, and with curiosity instead of recrimination (and also at the roots of the culture's problems—bravely, frequently, and with curiosity instead of recrimination)—that is, once you begin to work in the dark, and see in the dark, without being quite so afraid of, and antagonistic towards, the dark—what so often then begins to happen, slowly, down there, deep in the dirt?

You begin to grow.

Rather, you begin to grow *down*.

You begin to have stronger, healthier roots, and therefore a more solid foundation—physical, emotional, and cultural—on which to stand.

Which, I would say, is the prerequisite for growing up.

And that is very positive indeed.

But first:

You may have to poop into a tray.
You may have to quit or change your job.
You may have to ask for help.
You may have to say goodbye to bagels forever.

There is a reason there isn't a line around the block for this kind of medicine.

Hades sucks.

Embrace Hades.

That is the first step if you ever want to get out.

25

I think I had known for quite a while that this perspective change was coming, but like everyone else, I was clinging to the upper world for dear life. I just wanted my doctors to save me already. I just wanted positive pink clouds to levitate me out of there and deliver the miraculous cure I had been promised in wellness webinar after wellness webinar. I just wanted people around me to treat me the way they would treat any other sick person they knew—with dignity, and care, and respect.

Why was that too much to ask?

But the real kicker was, every single time that rose-colored way of looking at things did not work out, every single time the heroes did more damage, every single time people continued to treat me in ways that were hurtful and demeaning, and every single time the positive thoughts did not work—reader, I could not stop myself from boomeranging back to the message I had been programmed with subtly and unsubtly at every single step of the way:

The problem was me.

I was the common denominator.
I must be a very bad girl.

Up until Dr. Oops, I just could not stop myself from going there.

I should say: I could not stop myself from going there until I spent two years steeped in feminine and feminist literature. It really is not too grand to say that those women and those words changed me. They built a permission structure in my mind to do and feel as I had been wanting to do and feel, really for my whole life.

And so what a gruesome but useful gift it was to me for Dr. Oops to do an oops so flagrant, so violating, and then to try to redirect the blame at me (classic!)—right on the heels of that education.

I could now see this for what it was.

I could now see: this is just what they do.

They do the bad thing, and then they tell you that *you* did the bad thing.

And they do this because it works.

That is, they do this because it works for them.

Indeed, it had been working for them for well over a decade of my life.

And so reader, WOMI, whoever you are, I am here to tell you that if our sweet and sensitive protagonist has any hope of seeing the light of day again, after she has Embraced Hades and the onyx-colored glasses that come with, then she must, must, *must* take the next sequential step, and that is:

Reclaim Power.

If she is a woman, a WOMI, an HSP, or *any* kind of underground traveler, the world has likely taught her from the beginning to be nice, and compliant, and kind, and respectful of everyone's boundaries but her own. It doesn't matter what kind of violence, large or small, has occurred—most spend entire lifetimes accommodating and contorting and shape-shifting in order to please others, and simply do not know how—and do not have the support—to say no. And often, the person involved doesn't even realize it.

What tragedy.

So here is the thing. The way we treat women and WOMIs in medicine is a deeply entrenched and systemic problem—and deeply entrenched and systemic problems *do not change on their own.* Entrenched, systemic problems change because people make them change. And unfair though it may seem, those agents of change are almost always the ones who have been affected by the problem themselves.

What that means for the mysteriously ill woman is this:

If she is sick in the way that I am sick—with an illness of the shadow itself—then before all else, she has to understand that the experts, her friends, and her family are not awake to her problem. They are asleep. They cannot see her yet. They are on one side of the veil, and she is on the other. They do not know how to treat her properly, and that is just the reality. And while it is not necessarily their fault, it does more or less mean that *she* is the only one who knows what's going on.

She is the only one who knows how she feels.
She is the only one who knows what helps her and what hurts.
Her sensations, her emotions about those sensations, her emotions in general—they are valid, and they have been valid this whole time.

However, as we have covered at great and good length, she is also Cassandra: cursed to speak the truth that no one will believe.

And while this is a horrible, terrible, no-good reality:

It *is* the reality.
It *is* what's happening.

And that means:

She has to claim this.
She has to claim that her reality is the truth.
No matter what anyone else says.

Which will probably be one of the hardest things she will ever do.

An illness of the shadow is largely generated by the culture itself, and so it upsets people when she brings what she knows up from the root system and into the light. Because what's wrong with her actually has a little something to do with everyone else, too. People don't like hearing about pain to begin with—but they definitely don't like hearing about pain if *they* are in any way implicated. No ma'am. They want pain to be fixable. They want *her* to be fixable. They don't want to hear that they, too, might need a little fixing.

Which is exactly why, if a system is broken, our injured protagonist's being nice and kind and generous and compliant (at the expense of being fierce and honest and brave and just) doesn't do anyone any good in the long run. If a system is broken—no matter how broken she is—what is most needed is for her to say: no. *Especially* if she has even a scrap of freedom and power—because there are so many people in the world who have no freedom, no power, and no way to repair their broken systems.

And my dear reader, if you or the WOMI you know are reading *The Lady's Handbook for Her Mysterious Illness*, you definitely have a scrap of freedom and power. And so you must exercise it.

Because here is the truth:

Almost all positive change starts with a negative no.

We like to remember people like Martin Luther King, Jr., and Gandhi, and Maya Angelou for their big hearts, their love, their hope, their poetry, and their dreams. But in fact, all three of these exemplary lives were lifelong demonstrations of a forceful, soulful, muscular *no*.

Powerful women say no a lot. Which is exactly why most women are conditioned in the opposite direction—to be pliable and accommodating, and to say yes to everything. Yes to the second shift, yes to taking care of everyone else, yes to all the products being marketed to us, yes to painful sex, yes to bad sex, yes to painful clothes, and yes to painful beauty regimens. Yes to antidepressants for all of our physical symptoms, yes to disappearing our anger, yes to leaning in, and yes to tolerating being the only advanced country on earth without universal health care and universal paid maternity leave. Yesses all down the line, even though so few of us genuinely want any of those things. The case is strong that if we listened to women's No— much earlier and much more often, and if women listened to their own No, and felt that they were allowed and supported in saying No (and asking for the things they really want)—the world would be a much better place.

And so for me, with a nascent Queen of the Underworld flickering and flashing and glowing beneath my skin, that is how I took my first real step back in the direction of the light.

I said no to just about everyone.

No to my very opinionated father, no to my very opinionated brother, no to my very opinionated mother, and no to most of my very opinionated friends—all of whom had very pressing and very important ideas about what I needed to be doing next to save myself from this terrible monster of illness.

No to the endless follow-up appointments with the Oopses and Anuses of the world.

No to more ill-considered surgeries.

No to medications I knew were bad for me.

No to everyone telling me to look on the bright side.

No to those who admonished me to just be patient and trust that eventually my doctors would figure it all out and save me.

And no to the twenty health and wellness newsletters that contacted me daily, almost always selling something, almost always in all caps.

Unsubscribe.

No thank you.

No, no, no, *no*.

None of these people had the right, and certainly not the expertise, to be directing my medical care.

I had that right.

And I had amassed quite a bit of expertise.

And I needed to claim it.

And oh my dear reader, as my righteous no and reclamation of power echoed across the land—lo, the skies parted, the sun shone down, the mares whinnied, and the angels sang!

Jk, jk.

When I said no, repeatedly, calmly, again and again—oh dear, I disappointed absolutely everyone. I let down those who loved me the most, which was exactly why I hadn't ever wanted to do it in the first place. It was painful when these people met me with doubt, and anger, and an open spigot of new plans, new surgeries, new medications, new miracle supplements, new shamans, and new doctors I should fly around and around and around the world to see. It was painful when everyone expressed their sadness that I seemed to be giving up, and they tried to remind me that I was a hero, and that they loved that about me, and why couldn't I keep fighting? Forever? And ever? And ever? And ever?

I thanked them for their concern. Truly.

And then I let them know that the time had come for them to listen to me, and to help me in the ways I was asking for help, or to kindly leave me alone.

And reader, some of them listened.
But reader, some of them left.

And as difficult as that was, it gave me something I didn't realize I was missing.

When I stopped trying to please any and everyone else, I realized:

I was free.

~

Now, it's possible that you have gotten the sense along the way here that in my spare time I hold forth on the microbiome and microglia and cortisol at every chance I get—and indeed, as I have grown stronger, I have begun to do that more often—but at the time, I was quite timid about what I had learned and what I knew to be true, even after a decade of serious research, even as my Grand Theory of WOMI was proven more and more correct as more and more studies started to come out. My saying no to these people and asking them to listen to me was the first time I had really requested—no, demanded—that all the people I loved do the work to get into my corner, to check their disbelief and their half-baked ideas at the door, and to do everything they could to see things the way I saw them. This was the first sustained effort I had really put into being forceful about advocating for my right to be believed, my right to be respected, and my right to be in charge of my own health without being doubted at every turn.

Even though I was exhausted beyond recognition, even though I was electric with emotions, and even though I was bleeding into a diaper on my bed, over the course of about a month I called a series of meetings with each of my loved ones, and I began with the basics. One by one, I laid out the truth as I understood it—the elemental facts in the tragically curious case of Sarah M. Ramey.

~

Fact 1: I Have a Neuroendocrine-Immunological Disease

This disease is (a) fairly modern, (b) poorly researched, (c) very complicated, and (d) mostly misunderstood and/or totally disbelieved by conventional medicine.

However, (e), there does exist a growing number of people who *do* understand it—and these people have demonstrated that the main problem in people like me is a central nervous system that is inflamed, due to a variety of underlying, interrelated stressors. This inflammation then causes real changes in the brain, which results in wide-ranging dysfunction in the nervous system, the endocrine system, the gastrointestinal system, and the immune system. And that means that any kind of additional stress has a very real, very profound, and very negative *physiologic* effect on my body—especially in my case on pain levels, energy levels, autonomic system functioning, and on the health of the gut. And that means that most invasive or aggressive approaches—no matter how well intentioned, no matter how much we want to do whatever it takes to make me better—may actually make me much worse.

This is a fact.

Fact 2: I Am Not the Only Person Who Needs to Evaluate Their Psyche

The severity of my pain, and particularly the pelvic nature of my pain, seems to bring out the worst—nay, the id—in my physicians.

This is a confronting fact, but a fact all the same.

Fact 3: Certain Lifestyle Factors Help Me

Nutrient-dense food, enough sleep, gentle movement of my body, strong social connections, regular doses of creativity and humor, as well as a functioning hope machine have always lifted me out of the worst times, both physiologically and psychologically. And these are not woo-woo ideas—they are all commonsense practices that support the nervous system, the endocrine system, and the immune system, and are also all backed up by a mountain of science.

But these things do take time, and effort, and intention to nurture and to get into place—and it is impossible to do this while still on the medical Ferris wheel of constant, painful, stressful appointments and procedures.

Fact.

Fact 4: Doctors Are Trained—in Error—to Prescribe Medications That Can Hurt People Like Me, and to Condescend to the Supplements and Medications That Help People Like Me

This is a terrifying dynamic.

For example, there are six supplements and one medication that have always, always helped me—however, all of my traditional doctors pooh-pooh precisely 100 percent of these choices, and tell me not to take them. And that if I do take them, they will have no choice but to consider me both a hysteric and a simpleton. On the other hand, opioids, muscle relaxants, antidepressants, antianxiety medications, and birth-control pills have always made me much, much worse—including suicidal. This does not matter, and my traditional doctors are irrepressible in recommending these harmful medications to me at most of my visits, despite repeated descriptions of how badly I react.

Indeed, the more I describe how badly I react, the more robust the case becomes for my simpleminded hysteria.

Anyone would be terrified to find themselves in this dynamic.

Fact.

Fact 5: I Have Done the Work

I am not a doctor, but the reality is that I have researched and come to understand this phenomenon more than the vast majority of doctors. And while there is much more to know, there is a model of medicine (functional medicine, and anyone whose work is underpinned by an understanding of the microbiome, microglia, mitochondria, etc.) that takes cases like mine seriously, and has a set of treatments and protocols that work for helping people like me get on more solid ground. And this model of medicine is not fringe. There is the Center for Functional Medicine at the Cleveland Clinic.

This to say, the science (such as it is) is on my side.

Fact.

Fact 6: My Case Is an Outlier

My story is typical in many ways, but unusual in others. While I have gut dysbiosis, endocrine problems, and immune dysregulation (all typical), I also had a very bad thing happen to my pelvic floor in 2003. While trauma is a normal and initiating part of the WOMI story, a badly injured vagina is not. And as I had long suspected, there seemed to be a real problem in my pelvis that required further investigation—however, every time I tried to get help with that inquiry, I ended up with an Oops, an Anus, or a Hyde. I obviously wanted to keep investigating, but I had to be very careful about whom I worked with—which is an unusual medical dynamic, to have to *assume* most physicians are probably going to do you significantly more harm than good. In your vagina.

Also, re: outlier, there was some evidence (high eosinophils, consistent positive response to antifungal medication) of an ongoing infection of some kind, which might also be affecting my nervous system.

And of course, also re: outlier, CRPS is literally the most painful pain syndrome on the planet—and has no cure.

All of these extreme factors combined to mean that my red button was always being pressed, and until someone found a way to address those stubborn, outlier, root problems, it might mean I would be permanently stuck in the stress cycle, and dysregulating the microbiome, and cortisol, and the microglia, and certain autonomic responses, no matter what.

Therefore, to greater and lesser degrees over time, I might be permanently disabled.

A sad fact. But still, a fact.

~

Presenting my case in this way illustrated to me a lesson I have learned, and forgotten, and learned, and forgotten, again and again, and that is:

Making the invisible visible can be earthshaking medicine.

See: #MeToo.

This report from the root system really is one of the main goals of going into the underworld.

And because my case was so complicated and so consistently invalidated and yet so invisible, it was *profoundly* helpful for me to lay out all the facts of my case as real and important—another map, janky and homemade, but a lot more accurate than "a patient in search of narcotics." As a WOMI, it can be very easy to get overwhelmed with the number of proposed theories, the number of recommended therapies and treatments by friends and family, and the staggering number of denials that what you feel is, in fact, real. The level of invalidation is truly omnidirectional, it's unusual, and it *includes* your inner circle and what would normally be your support system. And so laying out the facts as you understand them—and laying them out as real, and concrete, and not up for debate among the armchair analysts—can begin to reinstall the rug that has been pulled out from under you.

Because let us be very clear:

I was quite alone in considering my master list of facts to be "facts."

And when I presented my facts, sometimes dispassionately, but often through tears and while bleeding into the diaper on my bed— they were not met with open arms or applause. They were met with distress, skepticism, frustration, judgment, and resistance.

And this is the most important thing to understand when invoking the holy No.

Generally it will mean being unliked, unpleasant, displeasing, aggravating, soft, unserious, or annoying—perceived by others as difficult, bitchy, bad, deviant, or, of course, crazy.

And if you are suffering from the Curse of the Good Girl—oh this burns us, precious.

We want to be liked, to be nice.

But as Stephen Sondheim teaches us in my favorite musical, *Into the Woods*:

"Nice is different than good."

~

The wind now in my disagreeable sails, I knew that next I needed to chart my own plan.

Like Alice in the face of so many Dodos, doorknobs, and Tweedles Dee and Dum—all letting her know at every opportunity how bad she is, how wrong she is, how strange, and how weird—it is Alice's job to remain indefatigably Alice.

Likewise, it was my job to remain indefatigably Sarah.

And so I did.

I made an indefatigably Sarah plan, and I presented it to the committee.

~

Plan 1: Protect Sarah

Because I have a neuroendocrine-immunological disease, it would be incumbent on me—and anyone who wanted to be on Team Sarah—

to remove as many antagonists from my life as possible. Not with any ill will or drama, just setting a clear boundary. This would mean no more surgery for the time being, and definitely no more doctors who didn't understand this type of problem. No exceptions. Not until I was stronger. And that might take a very long time.

Plan 2: Kindness Would Be the Rule of Law

Kindness and compassion were not just preferred characteristics— they were required for anyone in the Sarah Ramey inner circle. This was a firm boundary, and I frankly lost a few friends over it who were obsessed with fixing me, or harbored lingering disbelief they could not conceal, or clearly believed that I just hadn't tried hard enough, thought positively enough, or healed my soul enough.

Those people had to go.

But this kindness boundary included *me,* as well. The part of me that was prone to guilting and shaming and trying to perfect myself, so common in the chronically ill, would no longer get to sit on the ruling council anymore. And my kind self, my compassionate self, my forgiving self—she's wasn't just "allowed." She was put in charge.

But notably, this Kind Self also included my most-helpful inner advocate, which is a nicer way of saying my inner bitch. I had been a little late to the party in coming to see that an inner bitch is a fierce protector by responding negatively to aggression and abuse, and that is actually very kind.

Plan 3: Stop Fighting and Start Fostering

In the time I would free up from not going to the doctor all the time (and likewise, not having to recover from going to the doctor all the time), I would devote myself to what had always helped me: a gentle gut-healing program, gradually expanding my diet as tolerated, getting deeper and more sleep, doing gentle movement every day, stoking the humor and hope machines daily, and rebuilding the most important thing I had lost in my extreme isolation: a community. This was going to take a *long* time and a lot of patience, and the acceptance of a different paradigm. No ferocious questing. No extreme anything. No going it alone. And most unpleasant of all, I was going to have to ask for help from my friends and family. A lot of it.

Plan 4: Get the Necessary Medications and Supplements

I needed to find a physician who would prescribe Diflucan for me again, and monitor whether or not that was helpful. I also needed to find someone who would prescribe the medication low-dose naltrexone (LDN)—a medication I had found in my research that is thought to slowly help in regulating the immune system and reducing microglial inflammation of the brain and the rest of the central nervous system. Both Diflucan and LDN are of course pooh-poohed by traditional medicine; however, LDN is one of the only promising medications currently being used to treat both ME/CFS and fibromyalgia, and Diflucan was the only medication that had ever helped me. Those skeptical doctors were simply not allowed to be my doctors anymore and could go pooh-pooh somewhere else.

I also needed to make sure I was regularly taking all the supplements I knew for certain helped my body—despite my doctors' telling me they were dumb and unnecessary. That said, I needed to keep it simple, and not take all the many, many supplements that friends, family, and the Internet constantly told me I should be taking. I needed to be careful to avoid repeating the Great Crash—which, let us not forget, was caused by taking the wrong supplements.

Plan 5: Partner with a Competent Doctor

I would find the smartest functional medicine doctor I could (or someone equally fluent in the microbiome, microglia, mitochondria, etc.) and make sure it was someone who would work with me who really knows what they're doing—over the long haul. Functional medicine practitioners—good ones—are extremely hard to find, so I knew this might take some time.

Plan 6: Invoke the *Whole* Serenity Prayer

I was the queen of metamorphosis and very good at changing the things I could change—and would continue to do so. But I desperately needed to work on acceptance. To accept that my case was a real mess, and I might be living with a disability for a very long time. And as much as it burned my heroic ego, I needed to ask other people to accept this as well. To stop expecting and pressuring me to get All Better and to Win. False hope was much worse than gentle acceptance, and I needed to ask for help building a life *with* my illness, not a life in permanent opposition to it. And if friends or family didn't want to get on board with that, I needed to ask them to leave me be.

~

I called my plan the Year of Radical Acceptance.

Passive in theory, active in practice.

When you reclaim power in the regular, mundane world, you claim the right to say no to things that hurt you, and the right to ask for the things that help you. This is more radical than it sounds. You claim the reality of who you are—not what you think you are supposed to be. And you accept that you may have to train people how to treat you, what to expect from you, and what you expect from them.

For some of us, this is remarkably hard.
Usually because it has been made remarkably hard.

And this is why it is so important to take that inner inventory down in the root system and start to work with boundaries based on what you learn. Your yesses and noes may be completely out of order, and arranged entirely around other people's preferences. Especially with this illness, for which there is nary a single boundary to be seen (names are boundaries, diagnoses are boundaries, support pamphlets to give to your friends and family are a litany of boundaries— all things that are missing for you), learning to build your own parameters for yourself and for other people is foundational. You need to build your own fence, with a working gate, and preferably some friendly shrubbery so your new boundaries aren't unnecessarily harsh.

So what will that mean for a WOMI?

It might be simple things like writing a letter to friends and family and asking them to make an effort to understand the illness, instead of hoping they will do it on their own.

It might mean making her own list of Facts and Plans to share with her support system.

It might mean making the dietary changes she suspects will help her, despite being worried that friends or family will treat her like a hysteric or a simpleton.

It might mean writing to the NIH and demanding appropriate funding for the study of the mystery illnesses.

It might mean that if (when) a doctor rolls his eyes or snorts when she tells him her symptoms, she turns to him and says, "Excuse me. Please don't speak to me that way."

Or it might mean refusing altogether to make appointments with garden-variety doctors, because the honest truth is that garden-variety doctors are programmed with the wrong algorithm and will very likely treat her like shit. Which is a huge waste of time and energy and money for *both* parties. That is just the truth. Instead, she may need to do some dedicated research, and ask her community for help and recommendations, and find someone in her area who will take her and her case seriously.

But she has to do it.

Because Plan 1 must always be:

Protect WOMI.

It will not be easy. It will make other people uncomfortable, especially if she has been accommodating them her whole life. There will be eye rolls, and judgment, and grumbling, and conflict. But learning to draw these boundaries with grace, and learning to speak up for ourselves, is really required work for people like us.

We must do it.
Kindly, generously, collaboratively—but firmly.

26

Embedded in the reclamation of power is the next key concept I want to lift up and out and into the light, one that in the process of reconstituting her disintegrated self I am fairly certain she cannot proceed without, and that is:

Get a Witness.

In the long course of this illness, it has become clear to me that suffering cannot abate until it has been deeply seen and heard.

If you read the stories of survivors, or people who have suffered terrible losses—losing limbs, becoming paraplegic, losing their entire family—who then go on to become positive, healthy leaders in the community, it can sometimes look like it has everything to do with their own grit, determination, and will. They must be exceptional people, we think to ourselves. However, if you pull back the curtain, you will almost always see the same scene. These individuals who are able not only to recover but to thrive are the ones who are surrounded by people and structures that allow them to be deeply seen and deeply heard. Whether it is by a church community, or aides, or nurses, or doctors, or physical therapists, a strong support group, or by a close circle of family and friends:

In every case, their story has been deeply acknowledged.

For these inspirational survivors, you do not pull back the curtain to find their doctors, friends, and family saying, *You're dumb. You're crazy. You're lazy. You're weak.* There is no record on repeat saying, *This isn't happening. This doesn't hurt. It's all in your mind.*

It's the opposite. The support systems for these people know it's their job to say, *You're so strong. You are an inspiration. We could never do what you do. We love you. We admire you.*

This basic encouragement is completely absent for the mysteriously ill.

And any cursory scan of trauma research will tell you: when you systematically disenfranchise and stop listening to the traumatized, the victimized, the suffering, *that* is when people become embittered, or addicted to victimhood, and overly identified with their losses and their problems. Often, one finds that this type of perpetual victim has not been compassionately witnessed by the people who matter the most. Instead, they have often been systematically unwitnessed by the people who matter the most. Not enough people have pressed a forehead to theirs and said, *Holy fucking shit.*

Indeed, this is precisely the problem with the New Age self-help world. The entire worldview revolves around taking 100 percent responsibility for your life, for everything that happens to you, and for your own well-being.

And clean and tidy as it sounds, this is just not how life works.

We are interdependent.
We need one another.
No one is 100 percent responsible for his or her life.
We all need help, we all need care, we all need protection, and we all need acknowledgment.

We all need to give those things as well, for sure, but we also need to be getting them.

And if you'll allow me, I think our underground myth can help us one last time to concretize this concept. I found another woman who writes about The Heroine's Journey, Chameli Ardagh—and her telling of the story permanently cemented my reverence for the function of witness.

It goes like this:

You remember Inanna, the Sumerian goddess who dove into the Underworld, only to be killed by her sister, Ereshkigal?

As the story goes, the reason the great goddess Inanna went down in the first place was to attend Ereshkigal's husband's funeral. However, Ereshkigal's husband was a fairly terrible god—an abusive husband, who raped and battered Ereshkigal while he was alive—and so not only was Ereshkigal suffering the pain of having lost her spouse, she was also reckoning with a lifetime of violence, rape, shame, and anger. Thus, when her sister, the brilliant Queen of Heaven and Earth, decided to come pay her condolences, Ereshkigal flew into a rage. Inanna was too light, too shiny—all the things Ereshkigal was not—and arrogant enough to think she could disobey the rules of the Underworld and simply come as a visitor. The rules of the Underworld stated that once you came down, you could never go back.

So Ereshkigal, in her immense pain and shame, decided Inanna had to pay a price.

She killed Inanna, and hung her on a meat hook.

Such a very sweet bedtime story.

But let's keep going.

In this rather grim story of stories, how would you guess Inanna was saved?
In the usual manner?
By a prince?
By the sky gods?
By her father?

Or maybe by her own mettle, pluck, and courage?

Nope.

After three days of waiting in vain for Inanna to return, one of her priestesses realized something was wrong. She had been given instructions to go get help from the sky gods if Inanna didn't come back, and so off she went to find them. But to her surprise, when the priestess got to the sky gods, the (all male) sky gods laughed in her face. They mocked Inanna for being dumb enough to go into the Underworld in the first place. No one did that.

Not to be deterred, the priestess then went to the god Enki instead—god of the feminine elements water and creativity—and Enki came up with a solution. After listening to the predicament, he scraped the dirt from under his fingernails and fashioned two tiny flying creatures who could be sent down to pass unseen through the gates of Hell. He told the priestess that these were egoless creatures, and he told her to just wait.

So down through the seven gates the creatures flew, finally coming face-to-face with the great and terrible Ereshkigal, who was wailing and raging and moaning—for herself, for her husband, and now for her dead sister on the meat hook.

And unlike most stories we have ever heard about of saving women—instead of bargaining with the monster, or tricking her, or killing her, or stealing Inanna away—what did the egoless creatures do?

They mirrored her.

When she said, "Oh my aching bones!"
They said, "Oh, your aching bones!"

When she said, "Oh, my pain!"
They said, "Oh, your pain!"

"Oh, my sister!"
"Oh, your sister!"

"Oh, my life!"
"Oh, your life!"

And this is where the miracle of the story starts to unfold.

Slowly, slowly, with each wound seen and acknowledged, Eresh-kigal gradually stopped raging. Slowly, slowly, with each emotion expressed and mirrored back to her, Ereshkigal stopped moaning.

Little by little, Ereshkigal was transformed, calmed, and healed.

And as the story goes, these creatures were called the Mourners. They did not try to fix, or control, or do anything but bear profound witness to profound, lifelong, ugly suffering.

And once she was calmed, Ereshkigal was so grateful, she offered the Mourners anything they wanted in return. Anything, anything at all. And so of course, they asked for Inanna. So Ereshkigal agreed to resurrect her sister, and off Inanna went, flying back up to the surface to be Queen of Heaven and Earth again. Not saved by bravery, or feats of strength, or achievements, and definitely not by a prince or by the slaying of the monster.

What she was saved by is much more simple than that, and honestly, much harder.

She was saved by witness.
Egoless, mirroring witness.
Mourning.

And is this not so very true of real life?
That we simply need to be seen and heard in order to move on?
That we don't want someone to sedate us or fix us—first, we just want them to listen?

And not just that.
Are we not right to want this?
Do we not, so often, have something valuable that *should* be witnessed?
That requires time, and patience, and real, deep listening?

This is one of the main breaches of contract between the modern doctor and the modern patient.

There is just no time to listen, and not a whole lot of interest.

And the same is often true for a WOMI and her circle of friends or family—who want so desperately for her to just be fixed, and don't want to listen to her story or her pain.

This dynamic always reminds me of a passage from the great Henri Nouwen:

> When we honestly ask ourselves which person in our lives means the most to us, we often find that it is those who, instead of giving advice, solutions, or cures, have chosen rather to share our pain and touch our wounds with a warm and tender hand. The friend who can be silent with us in a moment of despair or confusion, who can stay with us in an hour of grief and bereavement, who can tolerate not knowing, not curing, not healing and face with us the reality of our powerlessness, that is a friend who cares.

Amen.

It doesn't mean that fixing doesn't have its place, it just can't be the only place.

So for our dear WOMI, it is so important for her to open a window onto her life, and to surround herself by those who are willing to perform this service. Even if it is just a few people to begin with. Though it is extremely difficult, she cannot give up on finding doctors who will take seriously how difficult this is, or therapists who will really listen, or friends who know how to listen, or a support group online or offline where people understand her and are willing to listen.

These people *are* out there.

She has to find them.

And she has to ask the people she spends time with to find that egoless witness inside themselves, even if it is hard for them, and to become those believing mirrors, even if empathy is an entirely new skill set for them.

It is not asking too much.

During the Year of Radical Acceptance, even though I felt embarrassed and sometimes ashamed, I was relentless about finding and sometimes teaching witnesses in my life. I just accepted that if I did not ask for it or seek it out or be willing to demonstrate it, it did not happen. If I didn't open the window, nobody opened it for me. I made an extremely concerted effort to make sure my family, my doctor, my friends, and a therapist saw what was happening, saw what approaches did and did not work, and saw that I needed a different kind of help than they were accustomed to giving.

This meant having a lot of conversations, often multiple conversations with the same people, to keep teaching them about what was going on, and what I needed, and what kind of responses were medicine versus what kind of responses were poison—all of which took a lot of effort, a lot of tears, and a lot of time.

But that growing acceptance of me as a valid entity—and a demonstrated willingness to keep working with me indefinitely as we slowly worked toward unraveling the mess—had a very real effect on me. It allowed my body and my brain to begin relaxing and to move out of their permanent position of terrified defense against the legions and hordes of naysayers.

It was not easy to have these messy conversations, over and over again.

And I still have to do it, all the time.

But it is always worth it.

So please, for you or the WOMI in your life, never underestimate the power of having a space held for suffering. Witness has a deep, almost mechanical function in the psyche. That box has to be checked, especially for the modern WOMI, in order to move on. It is not an indulgence, and it's not victimhood, for goodness sake. It's just a request for basic empathy. And especially in a medical setting, that's what healers are *supposed* to do. Witness has long been understood to be a key component of healing—but alas, time is money, money is time, and witness has come into short supply.

And because I know it may take her quite a while to find those many someones who will witness and who will believe, in the interim, if she is reading this right now, then let me press my forehead to hers and witness her myself.

Because holy fucking shit indeed, dear.

27

Okay, I know you're ready, but before we get on to some of the more strategic, dietary, lifestyle, and functional matters, there is one last mindset the average WOMI needs to install in order to make real progress, and that is:

Become an Ecologist.

These illnesses have to do with the *sum* of our many modern behaviors and environmental factors—not just one virus, not just one pesticide, and not just one evil company that leaked hexavalent chromium into the Hinkley water supply.

These illnesses are ecological in their nature.

While certain medications and treatment can be very helpful, and we do need to support those labs and scientists who are researching drugs that can help to turn off the worst of our symptoms, it is very clear that the mystery illnesses are not caused by a single, virulent, odious villain. The mystery illnesses don't come from one bad turn of the genetic roulette wheel. Like most chronic disease, they grow from the ground up.

Indeed, it is probably not a bridge too far to say that the mystery illnesses are like the climate change of the human body. A slow but determined man-made catastrophe.

Just like the drivers of climate change, the drivers of the mystery illnesses are complex, and multi-factorial, and generated by the culture—not by one bad actor.

Just like the symptoms of climate change, the symptoms of the mystery illnesses are complex and wide-ranging and have myriad presentations—floods, droughts, thousand-year storms, record temperatures. Not just one melting ice shelf.

And thus, just like reversing climate change, the reversal of the mystery illnesses is also going to be complex, slower than we want, and will require a true grassroots, multifaceted approach—not just one law, one surgery, or one medication.

One might call these inconvenient truths.

Likewise, because the problem is systemic, the solution is about creating *systems*—not just silver bullets—that grow health, instead of growing disease. Like climate change, if you don't stop the clear-cutting, the toxic dumping, the fracking, and the unchecked use of fossil fuels, then you might as well not try to resolve things at all. Behavioral change is at the heart of reversing climate change, it is going to require systematic effort, and it is at the heart of reversing the mystery illnesses for good.

So in order to truly make progress with a mystery illness, a WOMI has to orient herself to her life as an ecologist orients herself to the environment.

Said another way, she has to think of herself as a gardener, tending to her plot of earth. Instead of fighting her problem, she is slowly figuring out the systems for her life (like cooking real food, getting enough sleep and movement, and using non-endocrine-disrupting products) that need to be in place in order to make everything work better, and work more sustainably.

This is what I would call the heroinic response to life.

Of course, *heroinic* isn't even a word, and our discomfort with a heroinic response to life is almost a caricature. We have all become used to putting things like sleep, healthy eating, exercise, and stress relief in the forgotten cubby of Yeah, yeah, yeah, I know all that (but will never do it). "Get healthy" sits somewhere on the to-do list between "Call the cable company" and "Pick up the dry cleaning." And of those three, it is probably the least likely to get done. But approaching it this way does not work because it treats getting healthy as an entity, a metric, a thing—a box to check. And it is none of those things. Getting healthy is a practice. It is braided into the entire day, from the way you safeguard your sleep, to what you make for breakfast, to the way you get to work. It is an interstitial, cyclical endeavor, one that can't be "attacked," or "fixed," or even "attained."

For me, if I could give my twenty-five-year-old self one piece of advice, at the age where I started to explore what was really going on in my body in San Francisco, I would have taught myself to go all in with an ecological response to my illness. Which was, indeed, my first instinct. To water my own roots. To be tender, compassionate, restful, and nourishing. To install a battery of positive, repeating inputs. I would have counseled myself sternly against hopping from fix to fix—especially extreme fix to extreme fix—otherwise known as having a bad case of the Willy-Nillies.

But I did not counsel myself this way, primarily because I would have had to vaccinate myself against that other, much more dangerous condition, Magical Pillthink—and that inoculation requires almost superhuman strength, in our current cultural context. We all just want to click the Buy Now button and have our problems solved immediately. Our brains have become nearly hardwired to believe that anything—love, health, money, power, success—is on the other side of a neon Click Here box. People, including myself, are near pathological in their default to Magical Pillthink—and the magical pill of choice usually just accords to whatever tribe you're in. Case in point, let's take the way the mainstream is starting to talk about the microbiome. There is probably no more complex system in the body that we know so little about—and yet, the microbiome is starting to be hailed as the Fix for all of our modern chronic illnesses.

Obese? Depressed? Tired? Anxious?
Take one microbiome and call me in the morning!

Ours is a Magical Pillthink culture conditioned at every turn to believe that if something is wrong, there is always a quick fix, and virtually *everything* has an Eat Me/Drink Me tag dangling. Even when the thing is an "alternative" fix, it's almost always just the same narrative as Pfizer, dipped in coconut oil, rolled in chia seeds, sprinkled with stevia, and swallowed whole.

Because cures sell.
And Hades doesn't.

If it were easy, we would all do it, we would all click here.

But it isn't easy. It is a process, it takes time, it takes support, and it takes community.

That said, when you do reorient from trying to fix your life to focusing instead on fostering your life—that is, when you focus on your roots—this is when you start to get stronger, and stop pinging from one miracle to the next, feverishly defending your choices to friends and family, never really getting anywhere. When you stop trying to fix yourself, you realize that trying to fix yourself is actually a very miserable orientation toward your own life.

Instead, the enterprise becomes grounding—one of building a foundation, with repetition, devotion, and care. You leave behind what doesn't work for you, and commit to what does—even if it takes an extra hour of effort and time, and a little bit of money.

Much like the way a gardener relates to her plot of earth.

But in this case, she's the earth.

28

Now that our WOMI has got her mindsets, she is going to need to hold fast to these.

As soon as she sets out, no matter how hell-fabulous she is feeling, she will encounter the inexorable pull of the Light Side. The promised cures, the misleading FIBROMYALGIA SOLVED! headlines, the neon book jackets, the perfectly ponytailed yogis doing impossible headstands, the glowing green juicers—all undulating in a golden haze, singing sweetly, beckoning her with their long arms made of kale and coconuts. Or the other version of the Light Side: deciding she's the Good Guy in this story, strapping on her battle gear, and going to war with the Bad Guy of dark and terrible illness—armed with extreme yoga, extreme diets, and extreme cleanses.

Hold fast, WOMI.

Now we are going to talk about the next step, which will not be a surprise but will definitely make you want to find something else you can Click Here, or Buy Now—anything but what I'm about to describe to you. Because our next step is:

Learn About Functional Medicine.

The reason we have to begin with the mindsets and not the diet plans is because you genuinely cannot talk about this new paradigm of medicine unless the reality of this difficult situation has been accepted, a sense of loss has been explored, an openness to change embraced, the ecologist's mindset adopted, the balm of witness applied, and power reclaimed. Only when that cyclic, humble, realistic, underworldly, devotional attitude is in place—then and only then can we think about the next phase.

The what-to-do phase.
The science, the research, the habits, the hacks.

And in my opinion the most widely available place with the full range of what a WOMI needs access to (the correct tests, the right nutritional and behavioral information, and a skilled practitioner) is currently a functional medicine clinic.

Thus, we are going to begin with an overview of what this experience is like, going through the general outlines and principles—and as I say, just encourage you or a WOMI to *learn* about functional medicine. I am not asking you or anyone to run out and try it, or become a convert, or a proselytizer, or a microbiome bible-thumper. This is less of a prescriptive conversation, and more descriptive conversation. Functional medicine is still in its nascent stages, and it is in no way perfect—in fact, there is much to improve. It is not yet covered by insurance (which makes it very expensive and inaccessible), not all practitioners are top-shelf clinicians, and like anything outside the bounds of conventional medicine, it is always in danger of perpetuating the worst of the wellness industrial complex—overselling supplements, fear-based marketing, and all-caps newsletters. It is also quite, quite involved. There is a *lot* of pooping in trays, peeing in cups, and spitting in vials.

But these flaws are not unique to functional medicine. My outstanding $60,000 bill is for regular medicine, not functional medicine. My substandard medical care has been almost exclusively at the hands of regular medical doctors, not functional medicine doctors. When it comes to marketing, the pyrotechnic circus of a Pfizer sales conference is the stuff of nightmares, putting any all-caps wellness e-mail to shame. And of course, for every cup or tray I've had to deal with in functional medicine, I've had triple as many scopes/tubes/probes put up/down/in my various orifices at the behest of regular medicine.

So the notion that functional medicine is flawed does not mean we cannot and should not talk about this model of medicine now.

We can and we should.

This is the only evidence-based model that is truly attempting to get down to the roots of these problems, for the *full* WOMI spectrum—from mild hormonal issues, to moderate gut dysbiosis, all the way down to the severely ill mystery patient.

Furthermore, this is almost certainly the prototype for the future of primary care, and definitely the future of WOMI care. Integrative medicine and certain specialty clinics for ME/CFS have already begun to incorporate the best practices of functional medicine like stool testing, gut healing, HPA axis testing, and medications for microglial inflammation—which is good. The name "functional medicine" is not what matters. The principles are what matter. I'd like to see integrative medicine subsume functional medicine, and then primary care subsume integrative medicine. Because unless mainstream medicine is planning on ignoring the science of the microbiome, ignoring the science of nutrition, ignoring the science of the microglia, and ignoring the science of stress (a plan that makes the underground monster's eyes glitter and glow), this is the template that is required if we actually want to help the chronically ill, not just make money off of the chronically ill by keeping them sick and heavily medicated forever. (See: Pfizer, see: glitter and glow.)

So to begin our introduction to Hades-medicine (root-cause medicine), we're going to need a guide, a Beatrice, a Virgil—someone more experienced than myself—and I choose the prominent and respected practitioner Chris Kresser. One of the best functional medicine explainers out there, he not only runs one of the best functional medicine clinics in the country but also produces an enormous amount of educational material for the public, all of which is helpfully and firmly grounded in scientific literature.

Let's dive in.

~

To begin, there is a simplified diagnostic construct Kresser uses to explain how a functional medicine practitioner thinks about disease.

The practitioner starts by looking at the patient's exposome—that is, the major things she has been exposed to in her life, from abuse, to a poor diet, to mold, to antibiotics, to infections. This is put at the center because this aggregate exposure is at the root of these illnesses—*aggregate* being the key word. That is, if she has a real sweet tooth but basically had a happy childhood and took zero antibiotics growing up, then she will likely not have had long-term dysbiosis and HPA axis dysregulation, and thus she is probably not going to become a WOMI.

But if she was sexually abused, put on several long courses of doxycycline for her acne as a kid, and grew up with sugar and processed food as the backbone of her diet, and she's an HSP—she probably *has* had long-term dysbiosis and HPA axis problems, and therefore has a much, much greater chance of becoming one of Us.

The exposome is all a matter of degree.
It all matters, and it all counts.
And it's all highly individual—everyone's exposome is a little bit different, which means that everyone's treatment is a little bit different.

So the first round of investigation is a deep dive into that middle circle. What has her diet been like, and what is it like now? How many antibiotics has she taken in her life, and when? Was she a vaginal birth, or a C-section (which impacts the infant microbiome)? Has she ever had Lyme? *Bartonella?* Epstein-Barr? Been in a serious car accident? Experienced severe emotional stress? Suffered from childhood abuse? Is she exhibiting patterns of PTSD, from abuse, an accident, combat, or rape? What does her daily movement pattern look like? What is her sleep like? Has she ever lived in a moldy home, or does she suspect she does now?

None of this is to shame her—it's just to get a measure of the amount of stress placed on her systems, a sense of where those stressors are coming from, and how much she's doing to alleviate that stress. The practitioner will also do a detailed intake of any known diseases, and of all symptoms—no matter if she has five or fifty from that long list we went through earlier. Functional medicine practitioners know how complicated and strange these problems can become, and she doesn't have to hide certain symptoms for fear of being labeled a hypochondriac. With this kind of practitioner, the doctor's default setting is generally belief, probably because a huge number of them were WOMIs and MOMIs themselves once, and they know that no one makes up hair loss, weight gain, crippling fatigue, and severe pain just for kicks.

Then the data that has been gathered regarding her exposome, known diseases, and symptoms will help the practitioner decide which tests are the most likely to reveal more about what exactly has gone wrong—and for the moderate to severe cases, testing is absolutely necessary. Not doing any testing is deeply problematic, and to be avoided whenever possible. You want as much hard data as you can get, from the best labs—and most often these will be based around what Kresser identifies as the eight root problems (pathologies) found in WOMIdom and chronic illness, which should be familiar to you by now. In his words, these are:

1. *Gut dysfunction.* Includes small intestine bacterial overgrowth (SIBO), infections (e.g., parasites, pathogenic bacteria, viruses, candida), low stomach acid, bile, and enzyme production, intestinal permeability, and food intolerances.

2. *Nutrient imbalance.* Includes deficiency of nutrients like vitamin B12, iron, folate, magnesium, zinc, EPA/DHA and fat-soluble vitamins (most common), and excess of nutrients like iron (less common).

3. *HPA axis dysregulation.* Includes regulating the communication between the hypothalamus, pituitary, and adrenal glands, and balancing the production of hormones associated with those glands (e.g., DHEA, cortisol).

4. *Toxic burden.* Includes exposure to chemicals (e.g., BPA, phthalates, etc.), heavy metals (e.g., mercury, arsenic), biotoxins (e.g., mold/mycotoxins, inflammation), or impaired detoxification capacity due to nutrient deficiency, GI issues, or other causes.

5. *Chronic infections.* Includes "stealth" infections by tick-borne organisms (e.g., *Borrelia, Babesia, Bartonella, Ehrlichia*), intracellular bacteria (e.g., *Mycoplamsa, Chlamydophila*), viruses (e.g., HHV-6, HPV), and dental bacteria.

6. *Hormone imbalance.* Includes hormones associated with metabolism (e.g., insulin, leptin), thyroid, and gonads (e.g., estrogen, progesterone, testosterone).

7. *Immune dysregulation.* Includes autoimmunity, underactive immune function, and chronic, systemic inflammation.

8. *Cellular dysfunction.* Impaired methylation, energy production, and mitochondrial function, and oxidative damage.

I've mentioned it's complicated?

But the reason for the complexity is fairly simple.

A nontoxic environment, a diet of whole, nutrient-dense foods, an internal microbiome-friendly environment, eight hours of deep sleep, strong social connections, and ways to relax that aren't subversively stressful (like TV and social media)—these are all normal, basic, human needs. And so when *none* of those basic human needs is being met properly over the course of ten, fifteen, twenty, thirty, forty years of your life, this adds up, and there is a lot that can go wrong. It's not rocket science. When you consistently don't give the garden enough water, enough sun, enough nutrients, enough fertilizer—or conversely, if you give it too much sun, or too much shade, or too many chemical treatments—you should probably start to expect that the garden is going to wilt, that there will be pestilence, and that you will not be reaping a bumper crop.

Thus, tests for all of these common issues will be done—Lyme titers, screening for viruses, stool testing, testing for autoimmunity, testing for mast cell activation, testing nutritional status, and so on—as well as some genetic testing to see if she has the genes associated with celiac, or NCGS, or Ehlers-Danlos, or the genes associated with poor detoxification (e.g., the MTHFR genes), or the genes associated with greater susceptibility to Lyme and to mold, to help home in on a diagnosis.

And then based on her test results, the practitioner will put together a protocol.

Which, you may be noticing, is not revolutionary.

Patient history. Symptoms. Tests. Appropriate protocols.

No rain dance. No crystal cave therapy. No canoe trip into the Amazon.

It's the same as traditional medicine, it's just that the history (the exposome), the symptoms (our monster list from before), the tests, and the protocols are all based on a different set of health metrics (pathologies), most of which can and should be understood as predominantly modern problems (problems in the modern exposome). When these are the metrics to measure (the microbiome, mitochondria, microglia, etc.)—which are so different from the metrics measured in conventional medicine—the methods have to be different, as well.

And in this case, depending on what the tests show to be the root problems, for most patients those methods currently involve some combination of a gut-healing regimen, treating any infections, removing any burdens like molds and metals, targeted supplementation, and, of course, a baseline introduction of nourishing, behavioral changes like a nutrient-dense diet, stress reduction, and getting enough sleep.

They way I look at it, it's like conventional medicine partnered up with a well-developed inner woman.

~

Now, for our WOMIs 4 and 5—our severely ill patients, who tend to be very difficult cases—there are more factors to consider. WOMIs 4 and 5 can't just go on a paleo diet, do some yoga, and take a few supplements—whereas WOMIs 1, 2, and 3 often can, with great results. Lucky ducks.

The WOMI 4 or 5 has so much more to resolve, and she should not be surprised if she has pretty severe problems in *all* of these areas. Remember, if the overarching problem is one of broken-down barriers, a dysfunctional gut, severe internal stress, dysregulated endocrine and immune systems, and uncontrollable hyperreactivity—there is so much that can be going wrong at once, each thing compounding the next.

I studied Chinese in high school, and my teacher used to look over my shoulder at my terrible character work, shaking her head, exclaiming, "*Tzao gao!*"

Which means:

"What a mess!"

And when I look at my own health situation, or that of any of the 4s and 5s I know, all I can think is:

Tzao gao.

It's just a big mess. Even though it's nice in theory that we have better tests to start getting down to the roots of these problems, these tests in their current form and current state of not being insured are time-consuming, expensive, and the subsequent protocols are elaborate and require near-total compliance on the patient's part in order to work.

But in my experience as one of these dungeon people:
I think it's best to just accept the mess.

Accept that a calamity has occurred, it has never been treated properly, and, like any problem left untreated for way too long, it may take real time to unwind—if it can be fully unwound at all. Though the positive police will have my head for saying it, a WOMI 4 or 5 may never get completely better.

For the severely ill, with the tools available right now, the realistic goal is not total reversal.

She might reverse it, don't get me wrong! I've seen it happen, and I haven't ruled it out for myself.

But that really cannot be the goal. It is wrong to give false hope, especially considering this family of diseases is so poorly understood, and so wildly underfunded. It is wrong to tell a person who can barely lift her head to drink her healing broth that she just needs to get into yoga, and wrong to tell the person who starts wishing for death the moment she opens her eyes in the morning—as so many of us who are severely ill have done, including myself, not that long ago—that the paleo diet is the cure she has been waiting for.

That said, what a good functional medicine program *can* do for many of us down in the lazaretto is to bring us back to the surface. Not always to full health—but freed from the prison where no sunbeam, no sound, and no person may enter without making us worse.

But please do take note: for the severely ill, these protocols need to be implemented with tremendous slowness and care. If she is a Difficult Case (like me), it is *very* easy to cause a crash (hi), and so she has to proceed with extreme caution, starting at small, pediatric doses and working up from there. She should not start a bunch of supplements and medications at once. She should not treat everything her tests uncovered all at the same time. She should expect treatments that work for others not to work as well (or possibly at all) for her, and expect to make adjustments. And I will say, if she's like me and her practitioner is *not* proceeding with care, caution, and slowness—she really must speak up for herself and ask the practitioner to slow down. She needs to set some boundaries and make sure her sensitivities are taken seriously. We all want to return to our old lives, healthy and vibrant, climbing mountains—and we want this yesterday. But we Difficult Cases are a special breed, one that can always find another trapdoor to fall through, so please trust me when I say that rushing the treatment is not worth causing a collapse. Her central nervous system is on profoundly high alert, and even when the treatments at hand are waving a white flag, her body may misinterpret them as a fleet of white naval ships, and suck her back into the hull, sealing the hatches.

So she may indeed need to treat infections, chelate metals, remediate mold—she just needs to take it slow. She may indeed be asked to try certain supplements and medications—but she needs to take it slow. She will have to make certain behavioral changes—but only as she's able.

She'll have to respect Beatrice, but make sure Beatrice respects her, too.

~

Now, if her tests show nothing, or are inconclusive, or if she is entirely too sick to even attempt a real intervention, there are a few other important options in the kitty. Indeed, these options are often used no matter what the tests show, because they help such a broad spectrum of WOMIs.

The first is a drug called low-dose naltrexone, or LDN. This drug is being used more and more, as it has been shown to be quite helpful across the board, from autoimmunity to fibromyalgia to severe ME/CFS. It is thought to have a regulating effect on several types of immune dysfunction, especially microglial inflammation. And because this drug doesn't work by suppressing immune function (most treatments for immune dysfunction suppress immune function and therefore cause an upwelling of other symptoms), there are comparatively few side effects. It does not work for everyone, exact dosing can be a bit of a challenge, and it is not a cure—but because this drug has been shown to dramatically help quite a few previously unhelpable ME/CFS patients (including me), as well as a broad range of WOMIs, it is definitely one of the top-line treatments that any doctor, functional or otherwise, should be considering for difficult WOMI cases.

Next, if she underwent a full battery of testing but no tangible Thing to treat could be found, this may be the time to start thinking about trying trauma therapy and/or a neural-retraining program to guide the brain slowly out of permanent fight or flight. For trauma therapy, there are many options, but the most studied is called EMDR, and EMDR-trained therapists can be found almost anywhere. For brain-retraining programs, two popular options are Annie Hopper's Dynamic Neural Retraining System and Ashok Gupta's neural-retraining program—both of which are slow brain-retraining programs that work with the neuroplasticity of the brain to rewire it back into a state of parasympathy and normal reactivity. This is essentially an intensive version of what yoga, meditation, affirmations, EMDR, and tapping do for regular people: they help us rewire our brains. And if she is one of Us, she definitely needs help in this area. Her brain has been under assault for a long time—and even if the gut is back to normal, the Lyme is treated, and the cadmium cleared, it is often still the case that the brain is now hardwired to be hypervigilant and needs dedicated help getting back to normal. That is, a brain that is wired to interpret everything as an act of war is now her primary internal stressor—and once that can be calmed, everything else resets itself. And especially if *she* suspects that this is the main problem for her (my experience is that people often know when their brain is the main problem, just as they know when it is not), this type of treatment is definitely worth looking into right away.

Then, finally, there are discussions to be had about the wide range of experimental treatments coming down the pike—and a functional medicine doctor is a good person to have this discussion with. Fecal transplants look like they might hit the market soon, which could be exciting, or at the very least, interesting. Some practices are trying more tech-based treatments that help rewire the hypervigilant brain, such as transcranial magnetic stimulation (TMS) or vagus nerve stimulation (VNS). Some are hoping to come at the same problem with a psychogenic approach—for example, using psilocybin, a psychedelic being studied primarily at Johns Hopkins. More and more people are being checked and treated for having a range of different issues in the spine—from spinal fluid leak, to craniocervical instability, to spinal stenosis—which turn out to be fairly common in WOMIs, and a few prominent patients with ME/CFS have gotten radically better from those spinal procedures. Others are anticipating a medication called larazotide, which is being developed and may help with regulating zonulin, which would speed up the healing of a leaky gut. There is a drug called rituximab, which depletes B cell formation, used sometimes for patients with autoimmune diseases and some CFS patients. There is a drug called Mestinon, shown to be useful in POTS, and possibly mast cell activation syndrome. There is a new drug called Ampligen, which shows some promise for immunomodulation. There is a drug many ME/CFS patients feel hopeful about called suramin, which is a drug that may turn off what Dr. Robert Naviaux at UC Davis calls the cell danger response, as well as a new drug being studied called Cortene, which addresses the maladaptive response in the limbic system. There are medications for those of us who have POTS to increase our blood volume, such as fludrocortisone. Some are using ketamine infusions and inhalers and creams for severe pain and depression. And then of course there is the ubiquitous antidepressant, which certainly can relieve some symptoms for some people—however, it's important to understand that antidepressants aren't the only therapy for WOMIs, certainly are not curative for most people, and (in my opinion) should really only come in after looking under the hood for dysbiosis, infections, needed behavioral changes, and so on.

The miracle pills really are all welcome.

Just because functional medicine takes a more natural, ground up approach than the average patient might be used to, medications *are* used when they are effective.

As Chris Kresser says, functional medicine is in favor of anything that works.

I think we all are.

We just have to keep in mind the bigger picture. When we look at the things that are working, from dietary change to neural retraining to low-dose naltrexone to larazotide, these things always revolve around the same principles:

Fixing dysbiosis and leaky gut.
Correcting nutrient deficiencies.
Retraining a hyperreactive brain, stuck in fight or flight.
Lightening the toxic load.
Treating infections.
Regulating stress, metabolic, and sex hormones.
Calming inflammation, and microglial inflammation.
Supporting the mitochondria, and supporting the methylation pathways.

And it is just not possible to address all of that for this hugely diverse patient populaation with one miracle drug or surgery.

A wide battery of things got us here in the first place, and so while we *all* support radically increased research and funding for the drugs that will help us get better, faster, I believe we need to protect ourselves from the temptation of believing that one intervention is going to press reset and put things back to normal, for all of us, forever.

~

Functional medicine has a long way to go.
In a few years, as it iterates, it will not be as complicated or as expensive or as intensive as it is right now.

And more elegant protocols *are* starting to emerge, making it easier and better for everyone.

As we keep our attention and our ingenuity and our dollars focused on the correct metrics, it is going to get easier, more streamlined, cheaper, and more accessible. And honestly, if people want to wait until then—reader, I certainly don't blame them. I can easily imagine a not-too-distant future where a WOMI goes to the doctor, and straight out of the gate she gets a fecal transplant, a round of transcranial magnetic stimulation, and a single dose of suramin—and that being an immediate jump start on the way back to health.

I cannot wait.

If I never see a paper tray meant for my own feces again, it will be too soon.

But for now, functional medicine is the available model that is actually addressing the entire spectrum of these problems. We know enough now to realize that these are the metrics we need to be dealing with, like them or not.

And this gets us to our "soft" recommendations. Because no matter what jump-start medication you get in the future, and no matter what you suss out as your greatest internal stressor, and no matter how sick you are—it is also clear that *all* of us need to be sent home with instructions and support about how to eat, sleep, think, and move in ways that both help get things going in the right direction, and prevent the same issues from creeping up all over again.

She has to resist the inner cynic that tells her none of that stuff is important.

Because it cannot be reiterated enough:

It is normal, not weird, to eat real food.
Normal, not weird, to get enough sleep.
Normal, not weird, to not be connected to a screen sixteen hours a day.
Normal, not weird, to have strong, regular social connections.
Normal, not weird, to move around and not sit slumped at a desk all day long.

Our current ways of eating and being in the world have become "normal" only in the last few decades—and they aren't working. They are making us sick, fat, depressed, lonely, and ashamed—and no Jolly Rancher, no doughnut hole, and no Dorito is worth all that.

And that brings us to the next step.

29

JERF!

That's the next step.

Just eat real food.

That is the first behavior a patient will be asked to change, be she WOMI 1, WOMI 3, or WOMI 5. Which is tough, because no area of health and healing is more charged than talking about our diet. I suspect that our dietary beliefs take up residence in the same part of our brains as our religious and political beliefs, and it is nearly impossible to maintain a sustained, rational conversation with someone in a different dietary camp than yours.

And yet, we must endeavor.

Because by this point, we all know something is wrong with the Standard American Diet (SAD). While people may not want to act on that knowledge, there isn't a nutrition scientist in the world who would disagree with the idea that SAD is indeed sad. And there's also not a nutrition scientist in the world who would disagree that we need to be eating mostly real food.

This is the same as Michael Pollan's famous credo: "Eat real food, not too much, mostly plants."

And that really is the simple, most important guideline that *all* Americans (and people who eat like Americans) need to hear—and need help changing in their lives.

This basically means eating like it's 1935—that is, eating a diet that looks more like it did before the food system changed so dramatically. That means fish, eggs, fresh vegetables, fresh fruits, fermented vegetables, whole nuts, whole seeds, spices, herbs, fresh dairy, fermented dairy, fresh grass-fed meats, and whole grains. To JERF means to cut out virtually all processed food, to eliminate most added sugars, and to avoid foods with additives that have unrecognizable names like "butylated hydroxytoluene."

Notably, the farther away you get from the United States, the more JERF is just a normal way of life. Which is because JERFing is not the radical suggestion—*SAD* is the radical suggestion, we've just become inured to it. SAD is by far the dietary anomaly in the history of the world, and it has not been an experiment that has turned out well.

Also of note: let us not conflate eating real food with shopping at Whole Foods. You can buy real food at Target, Walmart, Safeway, Shop & Stop, Trader Joe's, and Costco—and skip the eighteen-dollar bottles of white truffle oil, the eleven-dollar bags of kale chips, the twenty-eight-dollar tubs of maca powder, and the tiny twelve-dollar containers of cashew butter. Those outrageously expensive items are the main reason Whole Foods is also known as Whole Paycheck. When we say whole foods, we do not mean chia-maca-turmeric-truffle chips. We mean actual whole foods.

Now, does this way of eating come with some real obstacles for the average patient?

Yes, it does.

First, you have to learn the basics of cooking, which is a learning curve. Meal planning, batching, budgeting, delegating, and basic cooking knowledge—these are a few of the things you have to learn. But for both men and women, learning to cook simple, cheap, real food is an extremely important skill for maintaining your health, for strengthening your own self-reliance, and for bringing *down* the cost of food in your home. The good news is, for most people, cooking simple homemade food is less expensive than takeout, and much less expensive than eating at restaurants.

Second, you have to make the time. That's hard. No way around it.

But third, if you are a WOMI, you're sick! You either can't or don't want to put in *more* effort.

Unfortunately, none of those obstacles matters at all to a WOMI's microbiome, her metabolism, or her endocrine system. She needs to find a way to stabilize this pillar of health, even if she has to ask for help. Even if it takes her a long time to get her budgeting, batching, shopping systems up and working well.

Because the *reason* to JERF is not to be good, or virtuous, or right-minded, or thin.

The reason to JERF is simply because JERFing solves a huge number of these functional problems in the body. Real food does not have any added sugar, but it generally has loads of natural fiber, and this combination helps to balance blood sugar—and, as you will remember, balancing blood sugar is crucial for balancing hormones. Spiking and dropping blood sugar yanks metabolic and stress hormones around, and over time they become dysregulated—but this can be solved by getting the food itself to do the balancing act. In addition to that, real food is microbiome-friendly, because good bacteria like fiber, and bad bacteria and yeasts thrive in a sugary environment. Also, a real-food diet should include regular portions of fermented foods, which help to maintain a happy microbiome—and a happier microbiome means a stronger immune system, a stronger nervous system, and happier brain chemicals and neurotransmitters. Likewise, eating mostly real food greatly increases vitamin and nutrient density, as well as omega-3 fatty acid intake—unlike processed food, which is usually calorie-rich, nutrient-poor, vitamin-deficient, and high in inflammatory omega-6 fatty acids. Vitamins, nutrients, antioxidants, and omega-3 fatty acids help correct nutrient deficiencies, protect against oxidative damage, and help prevent inflammation.

You've probably seen all of these buzzwords before, and that's because they matter.

If you are nutrient-deficient, inflamed, dysbiotic, have a lot of oxidative damage, and your hormones are out of whack—you are not going to feel good.

It's crazy that we have normalized being overweight, sick, and depressed.

And lest this all seems too strict, most health advocates recommend a diet of about 80 percent JERFing, and leaving between 10 and 20 percent for pure pleasure and fun. Which still leaves quite a bit of room for indulgences, for some bread, some alcohol, and, if you insist, some Nutter Butters. This is where the infamous Cheat Day comes from—which has you eating clean for six days a week and then going hog wild one day a week—an easy way of making sure you are not feeling deprived, which is critical for staying on track.

The thing to stay conscious of is that we have this ratio inverted at the moment—40 percent real foods and 60 percent processed foods is the normal intake for the average American. It's become normal to eat a bowl of breakfast cereal that has the same amount of sugar as a slice of birthday cake—even though you'd never have birthday cake for breakfast every morning. Thus, "eating in moderation" is not good dietary advice. If you're eating 500 percent too much sugar (which is very easy to do when the recommended limit is six teaspoons a day), moderating your intake will still leave you with 250 percent too much sugar. It's important to stay conscious of just how much we've changed the human diet in only half a century.

And so for the average modern eater, JERFing is the remedy to a national health emergency that we need to address now. It's not just for WOMIs—it's for her kids, her parents, her partner. We know there's something wrong in the diet, and we *all* have to start changing it.

That said, it is not easy. JERFing requires clearing the obstacles we mentioned, and that can be tough. And for some people, it is virtually impossible—which never gets mentioned in wellness circles. For example, if you're living on SNAP (the government Supplemental Nutrition Assistance Program), you probably cannot make this work. We have a problem with subsidies in our food system that makes a bag of Cheetos less expensive than a head of broccoli. And so if you're on SNAP or are someone in a low-income bracket and you're thinking there is no way you can make this work, you are probably right. You can do your best, but what you really need is for the rest of us to fight for you, to lobby, to expand SNAP, and to change the food system itself. There are several pilot programs around the country in which doctors can prescribe fruits and vegetables—on a regular prescription pad—and low-income families can take that prescription and trade it for vouchers at local farmer's markets. The vouchers get that patient free fruits and vegetables, just as they would get a free medication that was covered by insurance.

Because the point is: the challenges we face with SAD are all challenges that need to be *dealt* with, not reasons not to JERF.

So now that we've gotten that out of the way, let's talk about how none of this JERF talk addresses the real questions regarding your health that are surely at the front of your mind.

But *Sarah*, I bet you are wondering.

What about gluten?

What about the GAPS diet?
Or the specific carbohydrate diet?
Or the vegan diet?
Or a raw foods diet?
Or the WAPF diet?
Or the paleo diet?

Are you going to advocate one of those?
Or, can you please, like Michael Pollan, scorn those diets, condemning them as fringe and fad kookery? Can you please lay to rest this dietary insanity, and put those extremists in their place?

I cannot.

I love Michael Pollan, and think he is right on just about everything.

But not about this.

Pollan has taken a consistent stance that it is illogical to take bread out of the human diet.

Which is totally true—for Michael Pollan.

The reason the paleo diet, the specific carbohydrate diet (SCD), the GAPS diet, and the WAPF diet have all become popular in the last decade is for the same reason.

WOMIs.

MOMIs.

Sometimes (but not always): HOMIs.

You may have heard me mention this once or twice, but if you are a WOMI, your gut is almost certainly in a state of disrepair—to the point of leaking, inflammation, immune problems, and moderate to severe motility dysfunction. Your gut is not like the average person's gut.

In fact, Pollan followed up his articles on gluten with an in-depth *New York Times* article about the microbiome—which was thrilling!—and reported in that piece that he got some testing done for himself, and has a *fantastic* microbiome.

This is so key.

Michael Pollan's fantastic microbiome is likely why he can eat bread with such abandon.

Because it is this—our intestinal lining—that is quite literally the dividing line between the stricter "fad" diets and the general, more commonsense recommendation to mostly JERF. If your gut is not yet seriously compromised, you are free to JERF at will, and this will probably do you a world of good.

And oh, what it is to be you!

Free and wild.

Wild and free.

Intentionally changing your diet, but at the end of the day *able* to eat anything you want.

But for the intestinally compromised, we are not so lucky.

Because what has gone wrong with us is *specifically* in our guts.

Not in our arms, or our legs, or our ears.

We *specifically* have to heal our guts.

And not all foods are soothing or innocuous to the human gut.

When there is ongoing dysbiosis in the intestine, with the accompanying inflammation and a possible leaking gut—in order to heal this (just like healing anything), the intestinal lining needs to be protected, it needs to be rid of infection, it needs to be dressed like a wound, it needs only the most soothing things to pass through it, and then it needs to be reinoculated. Which is much, much, much harder to control when the lining in question is the human intestine and not, say, the skin on your arm. Your arm doesn't have to digest every meal, every day, no matter what. And unlike the gut, you can put your arm in a cast, a splint, or a sling.

This is why disrupting the gut is such a big deal.

It is *really* tricky to heal, because it is on duty, all the time, and cannot be put on bed rest.

Which is truly the best reason to protect the gut and the microbiome in the first place. It is a beast to heal.

But if our WOMI is past that, and she knows she has dysbiosis and/or leaky gut—which she very likely does—then she has to go on a gut-healing diet.

And that is what the paleo diet, the specific carbohydrate diet, the GAPS diet, and the WAPF diet all do. They eliminate the same things a real-foods diet eliminates, but they also cut out grains and beans—because grains and beans are the most intestinally irritating natural foods we consume. This is nothing against grains personally, and grains are enormously helpful in different public health crises like a famine. But this public health crisis is fundamentally different, and most certainly not about famine. This public health issue is about damage to the intestinal wall. And grains and beans have coatings that make them more difficult to digest than other foods—that's why we have to cook them in the first place, to break some of that coating down. We can get into the technical lectin, saponin, gliadin, zonulin weeds another time—but whether you are sick or healthy, eating grains and beans will always cause a little irritation to the gut every time you eat them, whether you're aware of it or not—so if your project is *healing* the gut, those foods are not your friends.

In a world without wheelbarrows of sugar, cupboards of processed food, and IV lines of antibiotics—that is, in a world with fantastically healthy guts—grains would be much easier to tolerate. This may be one reason you don't see WOMIs virtually at all in the developing world. But in the developed world, where ruined guts are commonplace, grains are revealed for what they are: moderately irritating to the intestinal lining. Incidentally, this may also be why you see these problems slightly more in predominantly white and more affluent communities—because people in predominantly white and more affluent communities have better access to medical care, generally get better treatment by medical professionals, and therefore have a much higher likelihood of taking round after round of unnecessary antibiotics for things like acne. Then again, another reason this problem is more visible in whiter and more affluent communities may be because the only people really being heard, or who feel comfortable speaking up, are those we traditionally make the time for—that is, whiter and more affluent people.

Bottom line: if you are a WOMI, cutting out gluten (and possibly most grains and beans) has to be at the very top of your dietary priority list.

Okay, but what about vegan diets? Those are healthy, and those are pretty much *all* grains and beans. This is a really interesting question, because many, if not most, people I know who have gotten well on a gut-healing diet would prefer to have done it on a vegan diet. A vegan diet is more world-saving, a vegan diet is better for the environment, a vegan diet eliminates the profound animal cruelty we see in factory farming, and a vegan diet can have myriad health benefits, as well (as long as it is not a vegan replica of the standard American diet). And if grains and beans were not irritants to the gut, a vegan diet is probably what a functional medicine doctor would recommend—in fact, it's what functional medicine doctors *did* recommend at the very beginning, until there was better clinical evidence to show that a paleo-style diet was better for healing the intestinal lining. And while it is technically possible to do a gut-healing diet as a vegan, you would have to soak all of your grains and beans (soaking helps break down the saponins and lectins, and is how grains used to be prepared) for every single meal, for the entire duration of the gut-healing program—and even then, that would be less effective than just cutting the grains and beans out.

But I think we can ease some of the tension here.

People who need to heal their guts need a paleo-style diet.

Once those guts are healed, many of those people are able to expand their diets again, as long as they are maintaining a healthy, happy microbiome. And there is going to be great diversity on what expanded diets work for different people. Some people thrive on less meat and more whole grains—whereas other people will find they really thrive on a ketogenic diet, which cuts out all carbohydrates and relies entirely on meat and vegetables. There are a lot of different variations on what works, and part of the process is being willing to see what works the best for you and your body.

But the most important thing is that it doesn't have to be a perpetual war of Us versus Them.

It doesn't have to be paleo versus vegan.
It doesn't have to be bacon versus broccoli.

Indeed, a healthy vegan diet and a healthy paleo diet—compared to SAD—are *largely the same*. They both emphasize eating mostly plants, both advocate nutrient density, and both cut out processed foods. That's a huge amount in common, and once their guts are healed, people often end up somewhere in between, on a diet with the celebrity couple name Pegan.

But no matter what, ideology cannot trump physiology.

It's very hard to save the world if you're still exhausted and stuck on the toilet all day.

And the gut-healing diet is nonideological. It's not about being good or virtuous. It's not about saving the world. It's not about getting a beach body.

It is just about what works.

And if we dig a little deeper into the world of gut healing, this is where all of our other confusing trends begin to make sense, as well. Patients with autoimmunity often cannot tolerate nightshades—mushrooms, potatoes, eggplant—and need to go on the autoimmune protocol (AIP) diet, which is a paleo diet, minus nightshades and sometimes corn and eggs. That reality doesn't mean *the world* needs to cut those foods out—just these people. Other WOMIs are commonly sensitive to dairy, especially pasteurized dairy. Others can't eat eggs. Some people do better with very little meat, and tolerate nongluten grains. Others can't eat histamine-rich foods. Others can't tolerate FODMAPS (which, as we all know, stands for fermentable oligosaccharides, disaccharides, monosaccharides, and polyols). Others, like me at certain times in my life, are not able to eat solid food at all, and have to slowly, slowly, slowly be brought back on bone broths and pureed foods as the gut heals.

When the gut is disrupted, so, so many things can go wrong.

Each person's gut is disrupted in a different way, and so each person has a slightly different version of the general gut-healing diet that will work best for her or him.

Therefore, if you come across people on a very specific diet, you don't need to roll your eyes or make fun of them on late-night talk shows. You can just say, "Oh, they're on a gut-healing diet tailored to their specific problem. Good for them."

It doesn't have to be a war.

Us versus Them is a crippling mindset.

But lastly, precisely because it's all so hard, if a WOMI does suspect she needs to heal her gut, she will want the help of someone who knows the pitfalls, knows the common challenges, and can really guide her down the long road of rebuilding a thriving inner ecology. This brings us back to functional medicine, where she would be supported throughout the duration of healing her gut—with meal plans, specific stages, directions, shopping lists, and so on. Because she can't just cut out wheat for a few weeks and say she tried gut healing. That's like never seeing an oncologist, picking and choosing which chemo treatments she feels like going to, and, when that doesn't work, saying she tried the treatment for cancer and it just didn't work. Gut healing is a lot more involved than cutting out one food or another, often involves a hyperspecific diet for her and her microbiome, and also usually requires some targeted supplementation to treat the dysbiosis and help heal the intestinal wall.

Maybe one bright day in the future, we'll all get fecal transplants and call it a day.

So great, can't wait.

But for now, we have gut-healing diets. And thousands of people who have radically reversed the worst of their WOMI problems *just* by healing their guts. And a growing number of studies to back up what has been observed in clinical practice for some time—this diet really does help people. So, difficult as it may be, I believe the WOMI in your life deserves to have this viable tool presented as soon as she gets sick—not after years of suffering, being told there is absolutely nothing she can do.

I don't know about you, but I'd choose sixty days of a challenging diet, even knowing it might not work, over staying sick for another two, five, ten years of my life.

Anyway, I do hope these clarifications can help put out at least some of the raging fires in the diet debates.

There *is* a problem in the standard American diet.

We all need to JERF, a lot more.

And if we are WOMIs and MOMIs, we probably need to take extra care of our intestinal linings.

And the scientific community will continue to refine what people should and should not eat as nutritional science, testing, and personalization mature and become more sophisticated. (Not to mention when the large nutritional studies conducted are independently funded, not funded by Coca-Cola and Frito-Lay—a dystopian phenomenon that is much more common than you might think.)

But this should be good news all around. If you hate fad diets, and you are not sick—good news! You don't have to go on a fad diet. You can just eat more and more real food, and reap the benefits—for you, your family, and your children.

All we ask, for the rest of us who do need a special diet, is that you think about it and talk about it like you would think about and talk about any other important medicine—because that's exactly what it is.

30

Following the diet, we have the next unpopular step, which is:

Go Back to Basics.

Basic basics.

Sleep, movement, a nontoxic environment, and a well-nourished psyche.

If the WOMI is a 1, 2, 3, or even a 4, a huge part of her project is going to be slowly, thoughtfully building up a more and more solid foundation—which revolves around adopting a set of repeating behaviors: sleeping enough, moving enough, lightening her chemical load enough, and relaxing enough. None of this is radical, and she's heard it all before—but these behaviors do matter. They aren't soft, they aren't less important than 3-D printers and telemedicine, and she is not exempt just because she is sick.

But if she is a 5: don't worry. I cast a wide protective net around her. She needs help, not more sleep hacks. I get it. Exercise can often greatly exacerbate severe ME/CFS (called post-exertional malaise, or PEM)—which most health organizations will not acknowledge. That said, in my opinion she should not jettison these pillars entirely. While some of these things can be curative for the less severely affected WOMIs, gentle versions of these same principles still tend to help the most seriously ill WOMIs, as well. It's just that the effect is more of a buffer from an unremitting storm, not a fix. But I, for one, want her to have all the buffers there are.

So she can take what is useful here, and leave the rest.

Because even though these basic-basics are almost embarrassingly simple, the reality is that most people are not doing them. Who among us is sleeping eight hours a night, exercising most days of the week, using natural products, meditating for ten minutes a day, and nestled in the bosom of our community? Furthermore, once you've made a habit of not doing it, adopting these behaviors in your life can be quite hard. On top of that, each of these basic areas of human health is totally fraught with controversy—*which* diet, *which* sleep hack, *which* type of exercise, and *which* method of stress relief is the bestest, most perfectest, most cleverest.

But we at the school of Can't We All Just Get Along reject this.

The battle of the life hacks is clickbait health, and clickbait health is for the birds.

Functional medicine has a levelheaded approach here, based around one important concept called "bioindividualism." We also saw bioindividualism in the functional medicine workup, and in designing a diet that works specifically for you, and this is also why functional medicine is sometimes called personalized medicine. Bioindividualism means that because of a variety of factors—from your genes, to your microbiome, to certain enzymes you have or lack, based on ancestry, to your blood type, and even to your personality type—there isn't one diet, one sleep protocol, one type of exercise, or one mode of stress relief that works for everyone.

This is important to take in.

It matters much less what she does, and much more that she just does it.

Doesn't matter if it's Zumba, or yoga, or learning to use a kettlebell—all that matters is that she moves, frequently.

Doesn't matter if she takes melatonin, or uses a weighted blanket, or powers down her electronics by 9:00 p.m., or uses lavender oil, or drinks skullcap tea, or works with a practitioner who can help her—what matters is that she gets enough quality sleep, and does not give up on finding a way to make it work.

Doesn't matter which natural brand she uses—she just has to begin the process of swapping out her chemical-laden products for more natural ones over time. She has to take seriously that many of the ingredients she grew up thinking were totally normal have actually been proven to be endocrine-disrupting, carcinogenic, or both, yet they are very much still on the shelves. She isn't going to get to Zero Chemical, and shouldn't try (not all chemicals are dangerous), but what matters is that she makes the effort to avoid the worst ones—slowly and steadily—over time.

Use me as an example:

Starting with one squat a day, then two, then three, I worked up (over a *year*) to fifteen minutes of doing a free workout online most mornings. No more than that, often less. And whatever the workout was, I ignored the trainer's zeal and adapted it to my own ability. I never pushed myself, because doing it at all was the push. If I had to scale back to only a few squats a day, I did, and I didn't feel bad about it. I just did it, and I felt *a lot* better when I did. It didn't cure me, but that's not the point.

I also made sure I was asleep by 11:00 p.m., I turned down the temperature in my house, I had the app f.lux on my devices to block blue light at night, and I read a novel to fall asleep.

Over time I have slowly swapped most of my personal products for nontoxic ones, mainly using safe and cheap alternatives I can get at Target.

These all make a difference.
I still do these things.
When I don't do these things, I start to go downhill again.

Nobody can get it all perfect, it's not going to click into place overnight, and none of this is going to miraculously heal anyone. But that doesn't mean that these aren't some of the core pillars of health, and it requires real attention and dedication, over time, in order to stabilize each pillar the best you can. The aggregate benefits from a neuroendocrine-immune standpoint are real. You are removing some of the red-button pushers. And so what matters *the most* is that you don't sweep it all away, constructing a fortress of excuses around you—which is what almost everyone does. You know as well as I do that if we were talking about a medication, even if it cost a bit more out of pocket and was time-consuming to administer, if you knew it would help you, and it had been prescribed by your doctor, you'd figure out a way to make it work. Or if there was a type of dust in your air vents causing your diabetes, you'd find the money to have it remediated. Or if there were segments of the population that truly could not afford the treatment, which is absolutely true for all medical treatments not covered by insurance, there would be major advocacy campaigns to make those treatments affordable and available to those populations.

Because we know how to respond to acute problems—with hard, heroic medicine.

We do that very well.

And now we need to learn to be just as serious and just as resourceful when it comes to chronic problems, and the "soft" areas of diet, sleep, movement, a nontoxic environment, and a well-nourished psyche.

And speaking of the psyche, our same bioindividual and daily approach works for finding ways to switch into parasympathy, or the "rest and digest" mode of our bodies. Most cultures have parasympathy built into the daily culture, whether it's through meditation, prayer, siesta, or just tightly knit communities where breaks are taken early and often. In our culture, we take smoking breaks.

Again, it doesn't exactly matter what you do. Meditation has become popular here in the West, and it works well for many people—making them calmer, more focused, happier, and healthier—but meditation isn't the only form of stress relief, and it doesn't work for everyone. There's also knitting, gardening, spending time in nature, yoga, qigong, tai chi, journaling, music, dancing, nature, prayer, painting, drawing, potting—just to name a few. The main issue is that most of these things have been replaced by five-hour binges on Hulu and scrolling through Twitter—something I deeply understand and am seduced by as well, especially when one is very sick and can barely do anything else. But we do know that television and social media can actually be quite stressful and cortisol-producing. That data is in. The point is not to demonize TV or social media, it's just to say that in a very real, hormonal way, they can't be a *complete* substitute for nature, meditation, and/or making things with your hands. And just so we're clear: TV and social media really are a complete substitution at the moment—the average American watches five hours of television per day and spends two hours on social media.

You will hear me saying this over and over again, but none of this information is meant to shame a WOMI or to push her beyond her limits or to get her to be thinner or to make her virtuous or to make her good, whatever that means. Sleeping enough, moving your body, limiting exposure to endocrine disruptors, and doing things that help the body switch into rest and digest mode—these are all known to improve HPA axis function, and to get things going in a more positive direction, and this measure is really all you should care about. I know exactly how hard all of this is to do if you are sick—but I also know how much better most of us feel when we actually get these areas dialed in.

However, all that said, let's say she really can't do any of it—her insomnia is an unbreakable spell, exercise makes her much, much worse, and her hands are too swollen to hold a fork, let alone cook a healthy meal or use a pair of knitting needles.

Now we arrive at the most overlooked but most important form of stress relief to get in place, especially for WOMIs who find themselves living in exile:

People.

Because nothing nourishes the psyche like our connections.

Especially for women, the endocrine system is soothed by being around friends—laughing and talking and kvetching and kvelling.

Researchers at UCLA have shown that the primary way women switch out of fight-or-flight mode is to "tend and befriend," which is another thing you can observe in most cultures, where it's common to find circles of women cooking, quilting, sewing, and crafting. You see this in the West with the female book club, where no one wants to talk about the book, and they are just so happy for the group of women they get to enjoy.

We need this.
We need our community, and we need our tribe.

Indeed, several studies show that strong social connection is *the single greatest factor* in determining health outcomes, for both men and women.

The trouble is, tribe can be very hard to cultivate out of thin air—especially as an adult. And for the mysteriously ill, this problem is compounded exponentially. It is often the biggest hurdle of all, because even a good support group can be hard to find. And so because we are inherently isolated and no one understands us—way, way more than your average Jane—it is very common for WOMIs to begin a slow retreat further and further into their toxin-free, gluten-free, friend-free shells.

This is the single worst thing we can do for ourselves and our health outcomes.

Way above and beyond diet, sleep, and exercise.

So while she shouldn't *over*commit herself, what she wants is to create some recurring social contact that fills her up (even a little), with people who fill her up. If possible, a book club, a knitting club, a support group, a music club. Or if she is very sick, a request for her now nearly estranged friends to create a system where a different friend comes and just sits by her bed with her every few days. So many people she knows really would want to help, if only they had instructions. In fact, perhaps the smartest thing she can do is to take all the changes we have talked about—diet, learning to cook, movement, etc.—and find a way to do them in a community instead of all by herself. Find a walking partner, start a healthy eating club, join a community garden. Many birds, one stone.

And, I know—if the WOMI is a 4 or a 5, this can seem completely and utterly impossible. But to the degree she is able, she needs to rebel against the idea that she is destined to be a snaggletoothed, misunderstood hermit, locked in her bedroom forever. She *has* to bring people in—no matter how she does it, and no matter what works best for her—even if it is just through her phone or connecting to a supportive group on Facebook. And by the magic of technology, most people have the ability to do this now—most of us have the ability to find people like us with the click of a few buttons. We can, almost all of us, join a support group in person, or join a support group online, or post on Craigslist or Meetup or Twitter. Or we can ask someone we trust to reach out for us.

And just so we're clear: many of these efforts will be in vain.
Some of them will be humiliating, when people say no or don't have time for her.
She must not give up.
Like everything else on this list, creating connection takes time, repetition, tolerating failure, and trying again. It's cyclical, messy, and something to be cultivated without a tangible goal.

Personally, I am a do-everything-by-myself type, and one of my many allergies is asking for help or special accommodations. But in order for me to regrow, I knew that Human Connection was by far—*by far*—my biggest deficiency. It always is, for me. My toxin-free, gluten-free, friend-free shell is made of unalloyed adamantium. In my case, I had to *force* myself to secure the social connection part of my foundation—but over the course of many, many, many months, I did build a community around me again, from scratch.

And like I said, it was kind of humiliating.
I had to ask my friends to call me more often. I had to ask some people to come sit by my bedside. I joined some support groups online. I joined every mailing list I could think of in Tucson—music, arts, the botanical gardens, and even, by accident, a club for the elderly.

Humility, *humis*, earth.

And at first, this mortifying Community Campaign did not work at all.

Everything except having someone come sit by my bed involved such powers as "sitting in chairs" and "holding conversation"—two powers I had unfortunately lost along the way.

Nevertheless, I persisted.

I started a support group *for myself* comprised of some of my disparate friends on Facebook. Oh, how embarrassed I was to start my own support group, *but oh, how it helped me*. It reminded me that my friends were still out there, and still cared about me, even if I couldn't see them face-to-face. It gave me a space to communicate how I was doing, and a space for my friends to post Tim Riggins photos and cat videos to make me feel better. As a group, we would sometimes watch movies together on Netflix at the same time and set up a comment thread on Facebook, so it felt like I was around people again.

Like water for my parched soul, it was.

And then, as I started to get even the minutest bit better, I slowly reached out to the people I had met before things had gone to pieces in Tucson. Keep in mind, I did not know these people well. And in my solitary confinement, I had become more and more shy. And explaining my gyno-rectal-fatigue syndrome again and again to new people, you might be surprised to learn, was (and is) a genuine challenge.

But not doing it was not an option.

After three years of near-solitary confinement, my heart was on life support, and the medicine of Other People—of laughing, of sharing, of shooting the shit, of listening to their problems instead of wallowing in mine—this was the medicine I knew I needed more than anything I could get in an orange pill bottle at Walgreens. So piece by piece, I made it happen. I explained my sitting situation to these new people, and my inability to last more than half an hour— that is, I chucked my shame to the side and explained and laid out my very strange needs. And because human beings are innately good, these virtual strangers showed up for me. They would pick me up and take me for a drive, so I could ride with the seat reclined and get out of the house for a while. They would come sit with me while I lay on the couch. They found places around town that had couches I could lie down on, just so I could lie down outside of my house. They invited me out, even though I couldn't go, just to make me feel included.

Bless you, Stacey, Dan, Curtis, and Scott.

And as time went on—when I started to do even better—I started accepting those invitations. Even if I could only be there for ten minutes. I started going to those Meetup events, even just to introduce myself and then leave. And when the day came and I realized the pain had lessened enough that I could sit in a chair for a short while, in a classic Sarah Ramey moment, I joined OkCupid. Not with the intention of dating anyone—"Nice to meet you, my vagina is broken, I have a disease most people think is fake, and I can only stay for half an hour. But tell me about you, Doug."—just to get out of the house, and because I wanted to go on lame OkCupid dates and gossip about them like the rest of the world, dammit.

And all of this—all of these good humans—even that hilariously bad OkCupid date with the pet spiders—fed me more than any green juice, any paleo diet, or any gut-healing program. These humans kept my heart from being crushed under the weight of everything. Second only to starting the drug low-dose naltrexone, working hard to connect with these humans was the most important thing I did for myself on the long road back up to the light. Because even though it took almost two years, even though I had to schedule things into my calendar like "Go to Calexico concert for ten minutes," eventually those tenuous and disparate connections I had to work so hard to create slowly morphed into real bonds, and an actual network, and a functioning web of support. And what a tremendous relief that was, deep in my cells.

I had all the reasons in the world to make excuses, and to be graciously excused from the obligations of social life. I could have easily become Rameymodo, the hunchwolf of Notre Dame, crippled and locked away in the bell tower. I had the world's worst pain syndrome, I couldn't sit in chairs for more than an hour, my blood pressure dropped if I stood up for more than ten minutes, I was still participating in the Bowel Olympics every day, and I ran out of energy unnaturally fast.

That is a Get Out of Society Free card if I've ever heard one.

But to quote Christopher McCandless from *Into the Wild*, who scribbled in the margins of his book just before he died alone in the wilderness:

"Happiness is only real when shared."

My eyes still well up when I read that.

Reader, I abhor being the invisibly sick friend whom everyone needs to orchestrate their lives around—and yet, if I do not accept that I *am* an invisibly sick friend whom everyone needs to orchestrate their lives around as my reality, at least somewhat—well, then I don't get to see anyone at all. Because in the end, I am the only one who can begin building the bridge from me to everyone else. I'm the only one who knows what I need, and I'm the only one who can ask for it.

In the end, we must always remember what my friend Curtis told me when I thanked him for being one of the people who showed up for me in the worst of times:

"Sarah," he said. "No woman is a wo-island."

And reader, isn't that the truth.

31

So, listen.

I can feel your discomfort.

I can feel the squirming.

I can feel the fuck yous and the resistance to thinking any of this health bullshit matters, be you WOMI or be you FWOMI.

I completely understand, and I greet you with compassion at the black gate.

Change is not easy.

Feeling implicated sucks.

It would all just be much better if we could either pretend this is not happening or hang our hopes on a cure, make fun of healthy behaviors, stick our heads in the sand, and valiantly suffer as we wait for the NIH to do the right thing.

But that is just not what the science of these illnesses teaches us.

The science of these illnesses, along with the growing stories of people who have gotten better, or at least somewhat better, all support the principles we find in functional medicine—we have to heal the gut, change our behaviors back into normal human behaviors, and usually take some supplements and medications (but only in addition to the rest of the strong, rebuilt foundation).

And because of this, I think it might be useful to give you an example of what a functional medicine experience and action plan might look like in practice—to remind you that virtually no one has escaped the age of SAD or the age of antibiotics or the age of being Always On.

None of this is anyone's fault.

And to prove it, let's take a look at the most typical of typical WOMIs—a WOMI who had no idea she was walking down this path until she walked right off the cliff.

Me.

Let's look at what I told my functional medicine doctor about my own patient history when I sought him out at the beginning of the Year of Radical Acceptance. And let's look at the plan we devised.

Let's do some Grand Rounds.

Because when I talk about all of these unhealthy behaviors, it's not from up on some high horse looking down on a sea of stressed-out, sugar-addicted imbeciles.

That was me.
That was my life.
I am you.
I am her.

Which is just to say, a totally normal person.

~

I was the absolute mean, median, and mode of a kid born in the 1980s. Exceedingly average by just about every yardstick, I loved *Punky Brewster*, I loved *The Fresh Prince of Bel-Air*, and my prized possession was a Michael Jackson record player, which came with the *Thriller* LP and a single white glove.

And as I grew up, my life continued to unfold rather unremarkably.

I was a beanpole, with long brown hair and an unwieldy set of front teeth. My parents divorced when I was five, they both remarried, and I grew up in a blended family. This split and the intense acrimony that followed had a marked and very negative impact on me, but it certainly wasn't the only divorce on the block. Life went on.

Then in school, I was just, sort of . . . normal. I was a bookworm, I went to a community theater camp, I had friends, I had crushes, I sang in the choir, I was a good student, and I was always pleasant and always polite.

And physically speaking?

Why, I was the picture of health. I canoed on the weekends with my dad, flew kites with my mom, played soccer extramurally, rode a bicycle, went for walks in the woods, and was the captain of my high school volleyball team. My parents were doctors, so I was well attended medically, and any infections I had were neatly antibioticked in the bud.

It was only when high school began, right around when I got my first period, that I started to develop some nagging issues—pretty bad skin problems, some fatigue, a very painful period, and a distended belly. But everyone said it was nothing serious—normal teenage girl stuff.

In 1999, I would go off to college in the Northeast, where I continued my career in normalcy (or more accurately, privileged normalcy). I did well in school, I sang in an a cappella group, I wrote for the school paper, and I sang in a very loud rock band. I worked hard, and I played hard.

Then, as we well know, at the age of twenty-one I suffered an unfortunate botched urologic surgery, and life would never be normal again.

~

This is the patient history collected again and again by most of my regular doctors along the way, and also by a new doctor, Dr. Functional—a doctor in Virginia whom I sought out after Dr. Oops.

What did childhood look like?
Any major illnesses?
Any history of major illnesses in the family?
Any history of psychiatric disorders in the family?

Average. No. Colon cancer, breast cancer. No.

Just like me, my patient history pre-Damaskus was exceptionally unremarkable.

And prior to Dr. Functional, it was reported that way in my medical file.
Unremarkable.
That was the end of the story.

Except, of course, for the fact that it wasn't.

Here we find ourselves faced with a fascinating exercise I'd like to walk you through. You see, for every WOMI with an absolutely "unremarkable" patient history, there lies an extensive, subterranean, subtle, and invisible history. It's an alternate history—a palimpsest below the surface. This is the History Not Taken, and the History Not Taken is where two roads diverge in a wood—traditional medicine, well trodden and leading off to the right, and functional medicine, less traveled and winding into the woods on the left.

To gather this history, let's look again at young, almost flagrantly regular Sarah.

For example, what did young Sarah *eat* while she was watching *The Fresh Prince of Bel-Air*?
And what kind of sleep did Sarah get as she got older and busier?
Also, what kinds of infections were those unimportant infections nipped in the bud?
And what were those nagging, unimportant symptoms again?

And, just to check, how many antibiotics did we say she took growing up?

Aha. The palimpsest quivers.

Here is a summary of the History Not Taken for young Sarah Ramey, an invisible history that was there the entire time:

FOOD

For breakfast in high school, on an average day I could be found wolfing down Eggo waffles soaked in Aunt Jemima syrup, followed by a bottle of commercial orange juice, trying not to make a mess on the drive to school. And if not Eggo waffles, then Pop-Tarts. And if not Eggos and if not Pop-Tarts (and if not Eggos *and* Pop-Tarts), then Captain Crunch, Cocoa Puffs, Honeycomb, or Lucky Charms—occasionally substituted with Raisin Bran or Special K as a vague, healthful gesture, at the urging of my parents. For a midmorning snack, ravenous again, I would pick up something from the school vending machines—Twizzlers, Kit Kats, or Twix, washed down with a Coke. Even though I went to a private school, lunch was still the typical American school fare—pasta, bagels, sandwiches, Tater Tots, pizza and/or fries (french fries count as a vegetable, you know), paired with a Sprite, Diet Coke, or chocolate milk. When I got home from school, I might make a bowl of SpaghettiOs, or a Stouffer's pizza, or any other snack around the house—string cheese, Milano cookies, crackers, Goldfish, Werther's Originals, Jolly Ranchers, Doritos, or Oreos. My two households had what one could call a lax policy on food, and frankly, no one was around to raise an eyebrow. I had four hardworking parents. There were plenty of fruits and meats and vegetables around as well, I just didn't choose to eat them. I didn't know how to cook, and it was easier to eat straight out of a box, a bag, a wrapper, or a can. And to be honest, I don't think my parents could possibly have imagined just how much their little Hoover was snarfing up all day long.

Now, please notice: on this day of average days, it is already 6:00 p.m., and *not one piece of nonprocessed food has been consumed yet.*

Later we would have dinner, courtesy of an actual adult now home from a long day of work, which did involve real food—chicken, mashed potatoes, and salad. But dinner was for me a way station on the road to dessert—usually a very large bowl of ice cream with chocolate sauce, carried back to my room while I did homework. If I stayed up very late doing my work, I would definitely need to go down to the kitchen to refuel. Which is to say, balance the highest tower of Oreos I could between my palm and my chin, and head carefully back up to my room.

But here is the kicker: I considered all of this healthy.

Observe:

At least half the time I chose Aunt Jemima *Lite* instead of regular Aunt Jemima.
Sometimes I went for Diet Coke, instead of Coke.
I didn't eat a lot of fried foods.
And—abstention of abstentions—starting in high school, I didn't eat red meat!

What a good girl.

Technically speaking, I was not just average—I was following the governmental health recommendations. Carbohydrates made up the vast and expansive base of my food pyramid, I tried to eat diet foods sometimes, and I didn't eat fried food or red meat. I ate my vegetables dutifully at dinner, and got in a piece of fruit here and there.

And anyway, who cared?
I was skinny.
What other measure of health is there?
To my teenage mind—and to almost everyone's mind at the time—thinness was the only metric that mattered.

And when I left for college, this nutritional pattern continued full stride, with one predictable change, and that is: large quantities of cheap beer funneled from a keg, on top of which I was very likely doing a handstand.

SLEEP

I regularly got six hours of sleep or less, generally staying up late studying or gossiping or reading until 2:00 or 3:00 a.m. This pattern was the same in high school and college. I was proud of myself for not needing too much sleep (I was tough, you see), but most days I grudgingly silenced the alarm with a bang of my fist, dragging myself up at 5:30 a.m. to shower in the dark and get ready for school—and I would have to sleep heavily on weekends and holidays to make up for the deficit.

EXERCISE

As I said, I was an active child—an avid canoer, biker, swimmer, and soccer player. My volleyball team was nineteenth in the nation. But then on admission to college, I stopped exercising almost immediately upon arrival. I wanted to devote myself to working hard and playing hard—the pillars of university life. And in fact, if I'm honest, I developed a bit of an unspoken judgment about all those pony-tailed pearl girls running nowhere on their elliptical machines.

UNIMPORTANT SYMPTOMS

At age fourteen, at the onset of menstruation, a host of problems had appeared. I developed very painful periods (often doubling over in the hallway, much to my embarrassment), I had very frequent periods (every two weeks, much to my confusion), I had recurring yeast and other vaginal infections (which my gynecologist said was normal, but which made me feel bad about myself nonetheless), I had an inexplicably distended belly (which made me feel even worse about myself), and I had acne on my chest and back (which I covered up and felt deeply ashamed about, and aggrieved that I never once got to wear a tank top in high school). Beginning around age sixteen, I was also starting to sleep inordinate amounts after school, falling into bed for three-hour naps after classes.

I did go to the doctor about these concerns, but it was all attributed to adolescence and growing pains. Accutane, antibiotics, and birth-control pills were administered to manage these symptoms—

all of which caused new symptoms, and none of which provided much relief.

INFECTIONS

At the age of sixteen, I traveled to Costa Rica and came back with a large, suspicious lesion on my knee. Disgusting, to be sure, but treated topically with no problems and generally thought to be nothing. I also had giardiasis, a gut bug, which was treated with several weeks of antibiotics. And somewhere along the way, I had exposure to mononucleosis, aka mono, which is usually caused by the Epstein-Barr virus.

But then, in addition to my maggoty lesion, giardiasis, and mono, the other infection I had as a child was ... drumroll ...

Lyme disease.

Twice.

Bullseye rash and everything.

I have also tested positive for *Bartonella* since 2003, bacteria that cause one of the most common coinfections that travel with Lyme disease—but in traditional medicine, this is considered an unimportant finding that does not mean anything and does not need to be treated.

But in any case, not to worry. At the time of both teenage Lyme infections, I was treated for two whole weeks with strong antibiotics—the standard course of treatment for Lyme disease in regular medicine. And I don't test positive for Lyme anymore—so it doesn't matter!

ANTIBIOTICS

Lastly, as you can tell, I took a tremendous load of antibiotics—regularly.

I took them for long periods of time for my skin problems (doc-

tor's orders), for the Lyme both times (doctor's orders), sometimes
for the gynecological issues (doctor's orders), and I took them for
any sore throat, any cough, and for almost any cold (often just at my
request—a doctor's daughter has almost unlimited access to antibiotics). And of course, I took antibiotics for six months for the PUTI
in college—and then *intravenously for a month* after the sepsis, on
some of the most powerful antibiotics that exist. And then orally for
eight straight months after that.

Because as was thought at the time—it couldn't hurt.

~

Now these are bombs I am dropping on you here in the eleventh
hour to prove a point.

Patient history is supposed to be taken seriously at the beginning, not the end.

But it wasn't.

At every single one of my conventional medical appointments, lo
these thousands of years as a patient—at the neurologist, the urologist, the gynecologist, the gastroenterologist, the infectious disease
specialist, the cardiologist, the rheumatologist—I told every single
doctor that I had taken a lot of antibiotics, that I had had Lyme twice
as a child, that I had very bad menstrual periods and pronounced
fatigue in high school—and absolutely no one cared.

~

So excluding some of the outlier/wild card aspects of my case,
for the most part, I, Sarah Ramey, have the case history of a WOMI
that should be presented to medical schools across the country. Here
are the boxes, and if your patient is a WOMI, you will see them all
ticked neatly one by one.

1. A questionable and very Western diet. Extremely high glycemic, low nutrient density, highly processed and filled with chemicals, food dyes, aspartame, and preservatives.

2. Poor self-care. Very little sleep, very little exercise, overachiever syndrome, and very little stress relief other than the kind found shotgunned out of a beer can.

3. An HSP. Artist. Musician. Writer. Human warning bell.

4. Adverse childhood events. It has been shown that a particularly bad divorce and then pronounced and ongoing rancor, normalized as it has become, can affect children as a trauma—deeply and negatively. And, like any other trauma, it can have lasting physiologic effects because of real changes to the brain's fight-or-flight response, and the real effect that has on the HPA axis, the immune system, the endocrine system, the microglia, and the gut.

5. All the most common initial warning bells—bad skin, an unhappy gut, an unhappy vaginal biome, a very disturbed period, and some fatigue.

6. Many, many infections, including an unknown tropical guest. (This may have been the *Strongyloides*.)

7. Lyme disease. Twice.

8. Antibiotics, taken like candy.

But for the most part, this isn't considered an interesting case history.

This is Standard America.

But in our new context of dysregulated cortisol, inflammation, nutrient deficiency, microglia, leaky gut, and a disrupted microbiome:

This is the exact, clinical picture of a ticking WOMI bomb.

Or to go back to a previous metaphor, I was moving slowly down the conveyor belt, edging toward the drop-off, totally unbeknownst to anyone. So now when we ask ourselves that original question—How on earth did this young girl suddenly become so mysteriously sick after a botched urologic surgery and an onslaught of antibiotics?— knowing what we know now, the real question should be:

How could she not?

This is why the History Not Taken is so important and must be incorporated into the training of future physicians. This is why being educated about nutrition, cortisol, microglia, the microbiome, and certain infections like Lyme is not just a nice idea—this education is the hook on which everything hangs. This case history is extremely similar to that of the rest of the WOMI sisterhood (and the smaller MOMI brotherhood)—because who didn't grow up on the standard American diet, viewing stress and busyness as a badge of honor, and mostly hiding their shameful symptoms associated with menstruation, poop, acne, and fatigue?

But without that palimpsest, all you've got is a normal young girl who used to like canoeing and flying kites on the weekends but is now a disheveled mess claiming without proof to be sick—acting out her pitiable melodrama, "like so many other young women her age."

I may be practically imperfect in every other way, but as an example of the most comprehensive, typical presentation of the modern WOMI:

I am Exhibit A.

~

Dr. Functional laughed when he finished my patient intake.

"Here's a test: do you know what your biggest problem is?"

In the past, I might have said, "Candida," or *"Strongyloides,"* or "Dr. Damaskus," or some other entity that we could blame and, in a perfect world, eliminate.

But curled on the exam table in my day-muumuu, I just looked up at him with a weary, sidelong stare and said:

"Stress."

And Dr. Functional hooted with laughter.

"Yes! Do you know, no one gets that question right?"

~

Dr. Functional of course uses the omnidirectional definition of stress, and so we proceeded to test for those stressors (and remember, at this time I was in a full-blown, WOMI 5, ME/CFS crash and severely ill). And after we had done this full functional medicine workup—testing my stool, testing my genes, testing my cortisol levels, testing for Lyme, testing for autoimmune markers—my tests revealed what I could have told him before I arrived.

I had a real problem with candida overgrowth.
I had very low cortisol.
My inflammatory markers indicated an ongoing infection.
And the test they use as a surrogate for microglial inflammation was off the charts.

That is, I had:

Dysbiosis.
Major HPA axis dysregulation.
A probable infection.
And the exact type of neuroinflammation associated with both ME/CFS and complex regional pain syndrome.

The first thing Dr. Functional was interested in was the Lyme—as are you, if you are Lyme-literate. I was still testing positive for *Bartonella,* and when asked to take the Horowitz Lyme-MSIDS Questionnaire, or the Lyme disease symptom questionnaire, I scored a face-melting 140 points—treatment being recommended if you score over 46 points. And indeed, I do have many Lyme-suggestive symptoms, like upper back pain, recurring bronchitis (which began when I first got Lyme as a kid), myalgias, sleep disturbances, etc.

But the treatment for chronic Lyme disease?

A year of antibiotics.

I didn't know whether to laugh or cry.

Even my father, who had come with me to this appointment, piped up and said,

"But . . . but what about the *microbiome*?"

I was rather proud of my father in that moment.

Because he was exactly right—a year of antibiotics, in my case as a longtime gut-dysbiosis sufferer and a longtime collapser in the face of aggressive treatments, could be catastrophic.

And here we have Exhibit B.

Or an excellent example of what you'll remember as a Difficult Case.

There are a *lot* of unfortunate truths in my case. Clear data that something is wrong, but unclear data as to exactly *what* is wrong. An absolute willingness on my part to make any and all personal changes needed—but extreme and unexplained pain in my pelvic floor, extreme bowel dysfunction, and thus extreme and ongoing stress and virtually no chance of a gut-healing program truly taking root. All the markers of WOMI dysregulation, but mixed signals on what's causing the dysregulating.

WOMI 5s and Difficult Cases are often a bundle of unfortunate truths—arrows pointing in all different directions.

And this is exactly why we've just spent several chapters pains-takingly making the case for creating a strong foundation. Because in the absence of everything else, while it may not cure you, that is the thing that will give you some solid ground to stand on. The absence of a miracle cure should in no circumstances mean that these Difficult Cases don't still get treatment, compassion, and ongoing care. Or that they should be subjected to a series of difficult miracle cures and ace interventions, hoping one of them hits the bullseye. What the Difficult Cases among us deserve *first* (not fifteen years later) is the strongest-possible foundation, and a stabilized core.

So that's what we did.

The solution we came up with—Dr. Functional and I together—took into account some possibilities for aggressive interventions, but also took into account the reality of my actual body, rolled fetally on the table. The reality of a body that responded so badly to most interventions, and a body that was broken down, and weak, and dearly in need of a stronger baseline.

We came up with a hell-positive approach.

We decided to make a list of future treatments I could consider down the line—possibly treating Lyme disease and *Bartonella* under the very close watch of a functional medicine doctor, possibly trying a fecal transplant once those become available to the public, possibly considering an ileostomy if function never came back to my colon despite all other microbiomic and anti-inflammatory interventions, possibly considering some treatments for severe CRPS, like ketamine infusions (also under close and careful watch of a physician), and also, at my insistence, further exploration of what was wrong with my vagina.

But none of this would be done before seriously making an effort to rebuild the foundation in this young, seriously debilitated woman.

We agreed to shelve the aggressive treatments for a year.

For a year, we put in place a strong, baseline functional medicine protocol. A gut-healing program, focusing on getting deeper sleep, very minimal but dedicated exercise, a plan to connect with other people, and taking the medication I had been wanting to try, low-dose naltrexone (LDN).

In other words:

Exactly the plan I had already mapped out for myself.

And as I was sitting up to leave and get to work putting this protocol into practice in my real life, Dr. Functional stopped me and asked me if he might say one last thing.

"Sarah," he said, looking down at the floor. "A terrible thing has happened to you."

This statement alone made my lower lip start to quiver. He continued:

"But I want you to know that you need to hold on. We are getting closer and closer to a real cure for cases like yours, and even if my colleagues don't want to believe in this type of disease yet, those of us who do are making real strides—and I truly believe there will be hope for you in the next five years. What you're doing now is good—it's the basics of what we need to do for patients like you—and soon we will find ways to make it easier and more effective. But in the meantime, I want you to be proud of yourself. Given everything that's happened, you could have given up a long time ago, or become jaded and cynical. You didn't. That's something to feel good about. So just do me a favor, and hold on. Okay?"

I looked at him with my large, watering, lamplike eyes.

This was only the second time in thirteen years that a physician had acknowledged that I was actually suffering, only the second time a doctor had acknowledged my strength instead of my weakness, and only the second time someone in a white coat had offered me some realistic hope.

And as I lay there, Ereshkigal silently heaved and shuddered and shook inside of me.

And Dr. Functional, the Mourner, patiently looked on.

We were already forty-five minutes over the allotted appointment time, but he told me that if I needed to, I should go ahead and cry. He wasn't going anywhere.

And oh, how I did. And as I did, a *huge* tidal wave of relief flooded in again, just as it had in Dr. Wonderful's office. My entire body uncoiled, my terrified heart relaxed, and my gratitude poured out of me in a river of tears. Gratitude for the acknowledgment, for the hope, and for dealing with the *reality* and the shit of my situation. And this river of tears did not land me with a new prescription for Wellbutrin, but instead a sad smile from Dr. Functional, who knew very well that most of his patients had never been taken seriously before—and needed that, as much as they needed anything else.

It was lying there on the table that I again felt the feeling—for only the second time in my life—that instead of falling, falling, falling, or groping, groping, groping in the dark, someone had met me, torch in hand, and offered to walk alongside me on the path out of Hell.

Said another way, it was the first time in a long time a physician had actually done his job.

~

Thanking Dr. Functional, I left with my parents, and soon I was back in a rental in Arizona, putting the plan into action. I had needed to get out of my childhood bedroom at home, which was demoralizing and confining. I could work with Dr. Functional via Skype, and so, at my request, I moved back to where the air was warmer and I had a slightly bigger radius in which to live my own life. My mother helped me move and get settled, and then, as we had agreed, I began to tend to my foundation, patiently, every day. I took my medications and supplements (LDN, Diflucan, liposomal glutathione, turmeric, vitamin C, herbal antimicrobials, and probiotics) and, as described, I attended devotionally to how I ate, slept, moved, and thought. I went on a gut-healing diet again, I put blackout curtains in my room, and

I set a strict curfew for electronics. I did a small amount of exercise most days, I sat in the sun for a few minutes most days, and I made myself laugh every day by watching Monty Python videos. I got off the medical merry-go-round, I stopped interacting with toxic people, I did a short, daily meditation visualizing strength, and I brought as much healthy community into my life as I could.

Put medically, I attended seriously to the three, known, biggest drivers of a WOMIpocalypse:

Gut dysbiosis, HPA axis dysfunction, and microglial inflammation. The functioning of my gut, and the functioning of my brain.

Knowing that I was not trying to cure myself.

Knowing that I was almost certainly missing a piece or two of the puzzle, which would have to be revisited later.

Knowing that my only intentions were to secure the foundation and to make life as good as it could be *with* my illness.

Progress was very slow.

I felt bad that I had no dragon to slay, and no goal to reassure others with when they asked.

"Radical nourishment" felt a bit lame.

There was a long list of more tempting, more extreme treatments I could have been trying.

There was a lot of trial and error.

But instead of seeing errors as signs I was on the wrong path, or signs of failure, or sending me into self-flagellation or confusion or running for a new cure, I now saw error as a sign to dial it back, to be *more* nurturing, to let myself off the hook, and to try again when I was ready. As we had agreed, I didn't push, and I didn't rush. As we had agreed, I had to tolerate slowness and tiny, tiny incremental steps forward—and many steps back. And as we had agreed, I had to tolerate all of my friends and family looking at me as if I had three heads for thinking this heart-based, slow-health method would work.

But then, in the summer of 2015, after two solid years of being trapped in a bed and not getting better at all, and after six months of tending to myself like an old, arthritic, and yet very determined gardener:

I began to regrow.

On August 17 of 2015, I will never forget, I sat down at an open mic in downtown Tucson, Arizona—with my red lipstick, with my real-person clothes, and with my classical guitar held in my hands like a golden sheaf of wheat. And as I looked out at the crowd of misfits and songwriters and comedians, after so long in that bed, so long watching the sun rise and set without moving a muscle, so long trapped in my house, so long trapped by my body, so long not even able to sing, let alone lift my guitar—I could physically feel the message coming from all of my cells, loud and clear.

Life.
Muted, but warm.

The best message I have ever received.

And so I want to go back, and underscore this point for you:

The fostering, the nourishment, the tending to myself, the commitment to daily ritual, the trusting of my own feelings and intuition, the emphasis on connection, the willingness to change, and the acceptance and surrender to the dark aspects of myself, my body, and my psyche—these were all, as you hopefully well know by now:

The feminine.

Partnered up with my already ultradeveloped masculine. I was already a whiz at discipline, creating habits, measuring progress, quantifying what could be quantified, and fixing what could be fixed—but I had long needed to slow down, and exhume, and take deadly serious those other complementary and necessary values, which are so easy to lock in the cellar and throw away the key.

And even though friends, family, and doctors looked at me and my feminine-revival plan, for the thousandth time in my life, with a mix of skepticism and pity:

It worked.

After about a year of devotionally implementing everything in my plan, I came back to life. I started dating one of those OkCupid boys in earnest. I created a network of friends. I planted a garden. I started to record music. I wore clothes that were not nightgowns. I got my own groceries and cooked my own food. Sly, winking cheer returned to its rightful owner. And I started writing again, with a fire not commonly associated with chronic fatigue syndrome.

Not cured.
But much stronger.

Not the conquering hero.
But alive.

Not positive or nicey-nicey.
But finally, finally:

Hopeful.

32

Reader, I am still sick.

I am not telling you this story to gild the lily.

Building a strong foundation did not undo that I have been violated in ways that can never be undone. Or that I've had my entire
adult life stolen by an invisible and malicious leviathan, by pain that
has engulfed every moment of every day, and by a thousand doctors
who refused to believe me. No book, no boyfriend, no archetype, no
diet, and no good night's sleep will ever make up for that. Not for me,
and not for the millions of women and men like me.

Resilience is not glamorous.

But it is necessary, and if you've been initiated into the underworld, you're going to need it basically every day.

Because guess what happens after our protagonist secures the
foundation?

Surprise!

She does it all over again.

She dives into the inky mirror, again.
She goes down to look at the roots, again.
She knows it's going to be messy, and she knows she'll only make
so much progress, again.

She knows that this is not backtracking, but rather assessing what's still off, and what needs attention in order to make things better up in the land of the living, again.

And to do this, of course she has to summon the Gorgon, again.

It had been a year since I had returned to the scene, light green and fresh, after so long in the ground. I was grateful for my comparably meager abilities, and I was doing my best to enjoy them. I could be found out with friends, or sitting in a coffee shop—not often, but when you've been locked in a basement for three years, going out at all is truly thrilling. But as usual, I was also still in a crippling amount of pain—and crippling pain is impossible to ignore, or gratitude-list yourself around. The medication LDN had reined things in somewhat, and the burning that had spread to my entire back and entire abdomen and entire left leg over the years had shrunk to a still-terrible but distinctly smaller gremlin curled around just the left side of my vagina, bladder, belly button, and mid-spine.

A clue.

Because the LDN was able to calm things down by a significant margin, it became clearer to me that some aspects of the pain were changeable—but some were not. There had been one brief, mysterious, golden year in Maine in the very beginning where the pain had reduced by almost 80 percent—but then it had returned, and forever after that the gremlin had never moved, not once, not because of any intervention, not ever. It was locked in on the left side of my vagina, where it felt like the little fucker had clamped its jaws and would not let go. Everything else radiated out from there.

And from the decade of research I had done, that was simply not the nature of a brain gone wild, sending signals about something that was not there and not real—and certainly not the nature of a somatized daddy issue, mommy issue, anger issue, or stress issue. That kind of somatic pain is different—it morphs and moves and flares and abates.

This thing didn't move at all.

This thing I was describing was the nature of something mechanical, something acute.

I knew this, I just couldn't prove it.

I knew this, but every yoga teacher, every Rolfer, every EFT therapist, every crystal-waving healer, every pain doctor, every gynecologist, every doctor ever—well over two hundred professionals— had all told me it was my brain gone wild.

But yonder gremlin said otherwise, and I had a newly formed alliance with my gremlins.

I refused to see a new doctor, because I knew what always happened would happen again. I refused to subject myself to more demeaning treatment, or to subject myself to the wasted hours and energy spent filling out new paperwork, traveling to some faraway appointment, and going over my lengthy story yet again, only to have it all thrown in the garbage.

I decided that the only way forward would be to extract better care from someone I had already seen.

And in light of the circumstances, I also decided that a little light extortion was perfectly reasonable.

Dear Dr. Oops, I began.

You see, after the incident, I had never actually given Dr. Oops the business.

What had happened with him in the OR was a very clear case of malpractice, but the truth is that I am just not the litigious sort. I know this is frustrating for many onlookers of my case, but if you have only one bar of battery life, all the time, it's nearly impossible to imagine using it up in lawyers' offices and courtrooms. I was also genuinely afraid that reprimanding this doctor would cause him to poison the well with future doctors who might want to look at his notes. Since my number-one goal was to protect myself and what was my very fragile health at the time, I stayed almost mute at our follow-up appointments, and left town without saying barely a word.

But I regretted that, and it seemed time to get right with Dr. Oops.

In the letter, I told him about how I was doing better. I told him about the protocol I was on, and sent him some information about LDN. I told him that the pain had reduced somewhat, and that I was very glad. I told him that my overall health had improved, and that I was very glad.

And I told him that this was no thanks to him.

Line by line, I explained to him in detail the error he had made in communicating with me, and then in the operating room. I explained to him how the mistake had occurred, and that the other doctor had already agreed it was a major mistake. I explained to him how violating it had been for me. I explained how I now had to live with a radio implanted in my left butt, and a network of wires in my pelvis. I explained that I hadn't asked for any of it, that it had been turned off for a year and a half, and that it very much still hurt.

I shook as I wrote.

But then I implied that while this was all perhaps actionable from a legal standpoint, it could also all be made right once again.

I could forget all of it if he would do me just one favor.

The favor that I had sought from him in the first place, which was not actually a favor at all, but a service, a profession, a calling, a *higher* calling.

I would let all of it go if he would just sit down and take my god-damn case seriously.

Aka do his job.

I asked him to take half an hour, maybe even a whole hour, and apply his mind to my case. I asked him to pull down my file, open it up, go over it again, and just *think* about what could be causing such severe pain on the left side of my vagina, pain that never moved and only expanded, that had started right after a urethral dilation gone awry. I asked him to leave the theories of psychosomatization at the door, because those kinds of lazy diagnostics are offensive and sexist, and I asked him to instead think seriously, and solemnly, and as if my life depended on it, because it did.

He wrote back to me within an hour.

Jauntily, he told me that he was sorry I was unhappy with our work together, and that he was glad to hear I was better overall, and that it sounded to him as if I had a neuroma, and that he wished me the best of luck.

I sat there, blinking.

It had taken me two weeks to compose my carefully crafted, poised yet fierce, emotionally honest yet professional letter . . . and he just fired his off, right off the top of his head. The brush-off, yet again. I was so disappointed. I almost didn't look up the term *neuroma*, which just sounded like another term for nerve pain.

But then I did look it up, and all the air went out of my lungs.

~

• A neuroma is a benign tumor of fibrous tissue that grows directly on a nerve.

• A neuroma is caused by some kind of trauma to the nerve, frequently a surgical trauma.

• A neuroma feels like a clamp, pinched directly on the nerve itself.

• Neuromas can be extremely painful, especially if the nerves are in a sensitive part of the body.

• Left untreated, neuromas can progress into an uncommon but severely debilitating syndrome known as complex regional pain syndrome, or CRPS.

~

Feel free to throw the book across the room.

~

To make a long story short, I had someone drive me to a pelvic-pain clinic in Phoenix, and on Dr. Oops's recommendation, they did the test I had been requesting for almost a decade—a transvaginal sonogram under anesthesia.

And wouldn't you know:
There on the scan was a fairly large mass on the left side of my vagina.

A mass so big, the surgeon was able to feel it with his hand.

No one (including me) had done a manual exam of my vagina, let alone a sonogram, in over a decade because it was too painful, and I screamed too loudly every time anyone began. That's why I kept asking to have it done under anesthesia—a request that was always denied because they said that would be an expensive, unnecessary test, and it would be a waste of time for all the personnel it would have taken to staff the OR.

It would have been, and I quote, "an indulgence."

And so it was missed. A mass on the left side of my vagina, deemed the likely result of Dr. Damaskus's slipping, missing the urethra entirely, and puncturing the left side of my vagina by accident. The pain was then likely amplified because I also developed a parallel inflammatory syndrome of the central nervous system. The golden year I experienced in Maine was likely a combination of two things: the Diflucan reduced the dysbiosis in my gut, which lowered the central nervous system inflammation; and then having sex likely broke up the fibrous tissue while it was still small and plastic enough to be dealt with in such a down-home, DIY manner. Then as the dysbiosis returned when I went off the Diflucan, and the central nervous system inflammation increased, more fibrous tissue had grown back, and over time it had grown quite large.

I was scheduled for surgery to deal with it immediately.

And when the surgeon went in, what he actually found was a much bigger issue than a simple neuroma. What he found was a large, networked mass of scarring and fibrous tissue, entrapping *all* the nerves on the left side of the vagina, fusing the veins to the bone, obstructing blood flow, and blocking almost all lymph drainage.

"A butcher," the new surgeon said of Dr. Damaskus.

The nerves were so badly damaged that one needed to be taken out.

Four months later, they took out three more.

This immediately reduced some of the pain, the swelling, and the bowel dysfunction.

Which certainly makes sense.

Because there was an actual, mechanical problem.

And there had been an actual, mechanical problem the entire motherfucking time.

~

I have no words for the level of rage I felt when this was finally unearthed.

That I did not go full Dexter is an absolute miracle.

~

Also, just to put a flag in it: as far as internal stressors go, a massive fourteen-year clamp on five different vaginal nerves—indeed, the most sensitive nerves in the body—this is about as stressful as it gets. Instead of a new diagnosis that upended the applecart yet again, this belated diagnosis just made Occam smile and nod.

~

So this brings us to our last get-out-of-hell tip for you, for the WOMI in your life, for us all—and I think it is the most important one:

Listen to Women.

Shortened from the original, "Listen to Women, You Fucking Motherfuckers."

My case went unsolved for fourteen years because no one would listen to me, and the reason they would not listen to me is because I am a woman.

It really is that simple.

The data clearly shows us that if you are a woman and you are in pain, doctors do not take it as seriously as they should. And if you are a woman of color or in any other way marginalized—forget about it.

In my case, I have the quintuple whammy of having ME/CFS, pelvic pain, CRPS, postural orthostatic tachycardia syndrome, and very irritable bowels—all of which predominantly affect women. And it is blindingly obvious that this ratio is what leads physicians to believe these conditions are partially or wholly psychosomatic. There does not exist an analogue for men. There is no disease that predominantly affects men that we have collectively decided is psychosomatic. There is no disease that predominantly affects men whose research is considered an indulgence. There is no disease that predominantly affects men where compassion is withheld because the doctors just don't like the cut of your jib.

Whereas, this is the *entire history* of women's health problems. Women's health problems have never been taken seriously when they first arise. If she has no outer proof, and if the disease is not imminently fatal—this process of telling a woman that it is all in her head is the feature, not the bug.

That I found myself screaming into the void is no coincidence.

And while this should be enough to rouse us all to action, this problem with listening to women does not just affect women. If you are a man and find yourself being treated abominably because you have ME/CFS, I submit to you it is because you have a woman's disease. Taking that a step further, if you are a man and find yourself shamed by others, or shaming yourself for having or showing emotions—this is because you are acting too much like a woman. Taking that a step further, if you are a country, and you find yourself in a laughably hypermasculine situation, pouring hundreds of billions into military and defense programs while cutting education (77 percent of teachers are female) and health care (80 percent of health care workers are female) and the social safety net (literally called "the nanny state")—that is, if you find your country is so out of balance that it is starting to fold in on itself—well, you might consider that this is a direct reaction to the long-overdue rise of women, as equals, who are equally powerful, and are interested in such things as education, health care, and programs to support the most vulnerable.

The fear and loathing of the female of the species—especially when she has stopped being pleasing, and subservient, and nice—is real.

Alongside racial animus, this is arguably the core sickness in our culture.

It is unconscious, and we're all doing it.

The way my doctors treated me was not out of malice.
This contempt for women, and for the feminine, is below the level of awareness.

This default to making wrong everything that has the blush of the feminine—especially the dark aspects of the feminine, the difficult feminine, the feminine that requires us to descend and work and change at the root level of our problems—is something that we all do, women and men alike.

But it disables us.
It is an act of profound self-harm.

While it was more expedient for my doctors not to listen to me, and to people like me, to shuffle me and people like me out of the office with a pat on the head and an antidepressant—not by the tens, or even the thousands, but by the millions—in the long term, that kind of behavior has created a *huge* mess within medicine itself. Illnesses like mine and the autoimmune diseases started to sharply increase decades ago—but nobody would listen, and nobody would fund the research, and so no one could get down to the root causes. Now an estimated 50 million Americans have autoimmunity. One in two Americans has at least one chronic illness—and while some of this is due to people living longer, the growing number of children and teens diagnosed with ME/CFS and fibromyalgia and juvenile diabetes and obesity will tell you that this is not just about lifespan. And even when we *do* know the root causes of chronic illnesses like obesity and Type 2 diabetes—the diet, the microbiome, lifestyle—because that stuff is soft, and requires change, it doesn't get to be a serious part of serious medicine.

The result is that we are now the sickest country in the history of the world.

We don't have enough doctors to take care of the number of sick people we have on our hands—and doctors are so overworked, they're starting to burn out. And our health care system is a massive and unnecessary burden on the economy, on businesses, and on individuals alike.

If we'd just listened to women in the beginning, the corrective actions needed would have been manageable. We could have poured our research dollars and our entrepreneurialism into designing a food system that was healthy and supportive and sustainable, instead of pouring our research dollars into creating red dye 40, glyphosate, and butylated hydroxytoluene.

This inability to listen to women is devastating.

Often bad, but bearable, in the short term—but always dismantling in the long term.

And so it is my strong contention that in order to bring things right again, torque must be applied where the actual point of leverage is:

Women.

And this is where I think we get back to the crux of things, because learning to listen to women means learning to *understand* women. And learning to understand women means learning to take seriously that men and women are not exactly the same.

Mostly the same, don't get me wrong.

But not exactly the same.

And if we don't take that seriously, then women and more feminine people will always appear to men (and to women who are more naturally masculine) as defective, bad, hysterical, and wrong. The male body and the male instinct are unequivocally our baselines of normalcy. And so when women have a different stress response than men, it's not seen as informative and valuable and different—it's seen as weak or make-believe. When women have a slightly greater impulse toward seeking connection and community, this is not seen as a wonderful example of *vive la différence*, but as a trick of social conditioning, to be unlearned in favor of self-reliance. When women are more vigilant about their family's health than the men in their family, this is not seen as a valuable, necessary instinct, but as being the nervousest Nellie.

And this creates a vicious cycle.

When we demonize the feminine in women, we demonize it in men, too, causing tremendous imbalance for everyone. Then women end up demonizing the masculine in men as well, because we're pissed, and can at least wield the power of emasculation. Then men demonize both the feminine and the masculine in women even more, because *they're* pissed, and can at least wield the power of Power.

Tzao gao.

We have to turn this around. We have to be able to look at these differences, no matter how slight, and appreciate the value that those different, balancing responses contain. If we keep thinking that equal means the same, we will not be able to come back into balance.

Observe:

When we look at everything we have identified as missing in the foundations of health in this country, almost every last piece of it is what we have historically and pejoratively called "women's work." Food preparation, food selection, telling children to eat their vegetables, making sure everyone gets to bed at a reasonable hour, banding together with other women to get the job done, and the use of herbs in health and healing:

Women's work.

Women have historically made the food that magically appeared three times a day, kept the house clean and in order, shopped for fresh food, planned the week's meals economically, and tended to children by taking them out in nature, putting them to work, and sending them out to play. Women have also traditionally been the social coordinators of any given household, making sure parties are organized, church is attended, playdates are made, and annual functions are kept in place. Also, as we have noted, women are the ones who almost always push to make sure no one in the family is ignoring their health and make them go to the doctor.

And who is it in the current system who holds your hand and offers a kind word?

Nine times out of ten, it's the nurses, 90 percent of whom are female.

This is very important to understand when we consider the out-right scorn people have heaped on some very commonsense ideas regarding the foundations of our health.

That bias is not random.

That bias is an outgrowth of the bias against women, anyone who identifies as femme, and the attendant bias against the feminine.

And it is critical to remember, *women* have this bias too. Women have internalized this scorn, just like women have internalized so many other aspects of the patriarchy. Many strong, modern women often view *not* cooking as the ultimate symbol of having arrived. Many strong, modern women assure everyone else that they don't go in for all that soft woo-woo stuff of days gone past.

This is a huge mistake.

It doesn't mean women should do all the cooking—Don't! Reclaim your power! Delegate!—but cooking and food cannot become the enemy. It doesn't mean that women have to carry the load of keeping everyone healthy by ourselves—but keeping every-one healthy cannot become the enemy.

Women's work cannot be the enemy.

That has already happened, and if we don't correct it, we are doomed.

Women's work is not a pejorative, and it is arguably the most important work in the world, for which, lo these thousands of years, women should have been paid, recognized, respected, and protected. But instead, in the 1940s, when women began to move into the man's world of work, while this was earthshaking, important, and historical progress, it also opened up a big vacuum in the kitchen, a vacuum that was filled over time by profoundly bad replacements, like Tony the Tiger and Chef Boyardee. In my mind, it says everything that for many families, for many years, Mom was slowly but surely replaced by Ronald McDonald.

A clown.

And look what happened.

Our health collapse is directly tied to women moving into the workplace—and it's certainly not because women working is a bad thing—it's because no one listened to women, no one took women's concerns seriously when that huge shift occurred, and no support was given in the beginning from the government or from men to pick up the slack at home. It should have been. Then, and definitely now.

And here is where we get to the center of my main argument to you.

The feminine, the female, and women's work have to be put at the center again.

Of our policies, of our health care system, and also at the center of how we construct our own lives.

Remember, the underworld is only *depicted* as the journey down. It is really the journey in.

The feminine is the center of health, the interior, and it belongs in the middle. The masculine, in all of us, is meant to protect and defend that bright, vital core.

The masculine is *strengthened* by valuing the feminine and protecting it—and weakened by valuing only the masculine and protecting that instead. Men are *strengthened* by honoring their own feminine elements, just as they are strengthened by protecting and listening to women.

And this is not a wild idea I cooked up all by myself.

NGOs around the world have all recognized that in some of the poorest areas, where poverty had been all but given up on as a foregone conclusion, shifting investments to specifically invest in women (not giving the money to the all-male governments, or to the husbands, which had long been the tradition of foreign aid) has resulted in those communities starting to rise quickly out of poverty, as if by magic. Because what they found in study after study by the UN and by UNESCO was that when you gave the money to women, those women invested *90 percent* of that money into their family's health care, education, and nutrition. This is compared to the 35 percent reinvested in the family by the men.

Ninety percent.

We all understand the male call to duty—our military—and we fund that call to duty to the gills. If there is a war, we know exactly what to do, and have the most prepared, skilled, well-funded military in the world.

Have you ever considered that there might be a female counterpart call to duty? One that is worth protecting, and funding to the gills?

I have.

And I think:

It's health.

Women are the keepers of health.
Of our own health.
Of our children's health.
Of our partners' health.
Of our communities' health.
Of the health of the Earth.
Of psychological health.
Of spiritual health.

Women have been the ones growing health from the ground up since the beginning of time. The world's food has been prepared and administered by women since the beginning. All the great leaders that we write about and build monuments to were tended to and raised and fed almost exclusively by women.

What has been used against us—our sensitivity—in its strongest form is the ability to respond to something negative before it snow-balls into an uncontrollable problem. Our tendency to accommodate and shape-shift and mold to everyone else's needs is also our radical ability to *change*—in its strongest form, it is the ability to evolve, to transform, to shed bad habits, and to move on. What is considered soft and weak—our care, our nurture, and our ability to morph—is some of the strongest medicine there is on Earth.

It is time to invest in it, and to look to women to lead us out of this mess.

It is, from my WOMI's eye view, how we begin to create a virtu-ous cycle.

Which is why I am looking at you, reader.

Because there are a lot of you.
I mean *a lot*.

And I think that you are the lever of change.

I think we need to listen to you.

And if you are a reader who is not sick, or a doctor, or a man—I am looking at you, too.

Because you're the one who needs to start listening.

We're all in the same off-course boat together—eating, think-ing, and doing what everyone eats, thinks, and does. These chronic illnesses, these communications from the body—they are not here to shame us. They are asking us to *listen* compassionately, slowly, lovingly—listen so that we might change ourselves, which is the slow but sure way we can help change our community, which is the slow but sure way we can start to transform the rather grim situation we have unwittingly created. And when we start to look at it this way—not symptoms as aggressors, but symptoms as communication—not underworld as evil, but underworld as transformer—not change as a radical overthrow, but change as love—then we begin to see that women and the increasingly sick bodies we inhabit are all encoded with the same message.

Open the black gate.

It's the invitation down into the feminine change process.
It is the rather painful—but important—dissolution, death, and renewal process.
It is initiation into the Persephonean journey.

And while this call comes to men and women alike, I really do think it comes to women first.

And I think it probably is because of our bodies, our crucial sensitivity, and our inherent ability to change with relative ease.

Reader, what I am telling you is that there *is* a cipher.

The cipher is the female body itself.

The cipher is women.

We are the mirror of the Earth.
And what is happening to the Earth is also happening to us.
And if there is going to be a healing—in women, but also at large—if you ask me, it will almost certainly come to pass (if it comes to pass at all) in this one ancient, Babylonian way.

It's going to happen because of women.

It's going to happen because we spoke the truth—and we were believed.

And that is no silver lining, my friend.

That's the moral of the story.

33

Reader, I congratulate you at the end of a long road.

You have endured a lot of my story, which is not a fun one, and I thank you.

And with any luck, maybe you will take some of this advice that I have reluctantly added to your already heaping pile, and maybe it will move the needle. Maybe you will start to think about health and medicine from the bottom up, rather than from the top down. Maybe you will change your diet and your biome, and, as for so many others, the reaper will begin to release his grip. Maybe you will start tending to yourself, gently, and will feel some of the stress and the striving and the self-flagellation start to fall away. Maybe you will bring those in your community in, allowing their roots to wrap firmly around yours, sharing nutrients, propping you up where you are weak, so that you can all grow together. And maybe you will find one of the ever less-rare doctors who believes you, and partners with you, and is brave enough to walk next to you on the long road through hell.

Or maybe you will start to wade into the river at the gate, and then realize *Holy shit, this is hard!* and skitter back to the surface. Or maybe you're reading this in your day-muumuu, eating a piece of breakfast pizza, smoking a cigarette, thinking, *Fuck you, lady,* and wanting to hang me on the meat hook.

I congratulate you either way.

If you haven't thrown this book out the window yet (and even if you have), progress has been made. Because all I want is for you just to consider the information we know now about these diseases, and just to consider the uncomfortable possibility that we are a part of the problem—and the equally uncomfortable possibility that we are a part of the solution. Not because I want you to run out and heal the world tomorrow, and not because you must rise up from your bed in your gossamer robes and divine feminine glory—but because these changes are probably coming whether we like them or not. Nobody puts Kali in a corner. Demeter is wiping out life in the upper world, in her rage and sadness. And I believe that when these kinds of big, cultural changes come knocking, it is helpful to know why they're here in the first place, and to have some tools so that you yourself might evolve with more grace and less resistance when the day comes.

I think of this emerging team as the Reconstructionists.

The Humpty Dumpty Rescue Squad.

And you can see the need for this kind of team in just about every area of modern life. We live in an age of trauma, an enormous collision of ideas and nations and genders and religions and ideologies, and so it matters that we don't go running for the hills. And it matters that we don't become entrenched, reflexively, in a war mentality of Us versus Them. It matters that we roll up our sleeves, that we put on our Queen of the Dead hats, and that we get to work.

We need to change the American diet, and make real food affordable. We need to change the algorithm, and the way doctors treat the WOMIs who come through their doors. We need to pressure the NIH to do its job and properly fund the research for these diseases. We need to make rest, and connection, and nourishment, and empathy the new badges of honor. We need to tackle the addiction to short-term gain, and rebalance it with systems that support long-term health.

It's a lot.

Underworld people may lead the way, but there is something for everyone to do. Not everybody is a gung ho, hopemongering heal-ophile like myself—and if that's you, the more masculine, more skeptical type, let me be clear: you are just as important to the cause, and a powerful balancing force for me and my kind as we move forward.

For example, if you think all of this getting-healthy stuff is too expensive—instead of using that as an excuse to turn away, I would encourage you instead to lobby to have all types of preventative care covered by insurance (gym memberships, yoga classes, functional medicine, and even vouchers for fruits and vegetables), and for the government to expand our food-assistance programs like SNAP. Or let's say you're resistant to the paleo diet as a way to manipulate the microbiome—in that case, I would encourage you to support research initiatives to make fecal transplants easy and safe and available to everyone. If you're a doctor or a researcher who stiffens at the mention of a healthy diet and exercise, I would encourage you to take that energy and use it to demand large, controlled, well-designed studies about diet and exercise that aren't funded by Coca-Cola and Frito-Lay, so that the data we're all operating with can be sound.

But what you can't do is just sit on the sidelines and throw stones. Not anymore.
Like denying climate change, that time is gone.

And then, for those of you who can't do these things—that is, for those of you who are very, very, very sick:

Oh friend, we need you most of all.

We need you to make the invisible visible.

We need you to open a window onto your life, so that it is impossible for outsiders to pretend—as so many have, for so many decades—that you are not there. We need you to break the silence, even though the shame and the bullshit that will come your way are real.

We need you to do it anyway.

We need you to do it so that we may mourn you.

Because the more of us who do this, the more of us who bind together and speak up and take up room and make ourselves visible—at the risk of being disagreeable, and unpleasant, and unliked—the more powerful we become. And the more powerful we become, the more the gears of change will start to turn. This is how it works, this is how it has always worked—and this is already happening. Winter has been here for quite a while for people like us—but now you can see the first hints of spring. The advocacy is growing stronger. The documentaries are being made. The support groups are becoming more robust. The funding is finally beginning to move in the right direction. Because of the re-fucking-lentless work by thousands of people like you, the root system is getting healthier.

Not only that—this underworld story is clearly banging at the cellar door *everywhere*.

It wants to come up and through the whole culture.

Just look around.

It is a society that is shaking and trembling and in some ways crumbling, leaning unsustainably in a yangish direction, and the problem that has manifest itself in your body—it is *the* problem, and you are just one of a hundred million ringing bells. The culture is sick, and the amount of healing needed is enough to make anyone want to hibernate for a decade—which, of course, is exactly what most people are trying to do, and have done for a very long time.

And it's not that we need less heroism to deal with this, or less of that expansive entrepreneurial spirit that so defines the West.

It's just that we need more heroinism.

We need the people who have been forced to grow down.

We need—we have long needed—the return of the cultural mother.

We need the collective nurturer and caretaker and empath and the one who can see the big picture, who is fierce and slaps us upside the head when we're being foolish. Who demands that we have integrity, and close ties, and a strong foundation, and something good to eat. Who improves communities from the inside out—with education, nutrition, connection, community, and a repeating kind of work that has no real beginning and no real end.

We need this person more than ever.

And what I would propose to you, if you're reading this book about vaginas and poop and pain and despair and trauma and loss, and yet somehow you, too, still have that unshakable feeling of hope, of a way forward, of the possibility of healing, no matter how slow:

It's you.

It does not matter if you are a woman or a man.

The hero's journey has an ending, and so does its twin.

The way the myth of trauma ends, which is what I see playing out everywhere in a thousand different ways, in a thousand different people, is just like the end of Alice's traumatic story. It's just like the end of Snow White's traumatic story, and just like the end of Sleeping Beauty's traumatic story.

For what happens at the end of all of those fairy tales for little girls?

That's right, reader.

They wake up.

~

Along these lines, I have one last story that I would like to share.

There once was a physician named James N. Ramey, an endocrinologist and a medical traditionalist practicing in Washington, D.C. You'll remember him as the great pooh-pooher of alternative medicine, the prescriber of antidepressants, the loving but ultimately disbelieving father of your narrator. And while this narrator had always appreciated having her views challenged and refined, it had also been quite painful to be so at odds with a parent concerning the reality of her disease, not to mention the reality of her professional research.

And it had been equally painful for her father to watch his daughter suffer so badly, for so long, and to not be able to save her. He was trained as a white knight for just such situations.

But the truth was, all the people this narrator loved were eventually dragged into the underworld because of her situation. Because that's how empathy works—it opens you to another's experience, and it is painful.

But it has another function, too.

To allow yourself to feel with another, to go through what they are going through—is to open yourself to being moved, affected, shifted, changed, transformed.

It isn't just the sufferer who wakes up—it's the people who allow themselves to feel someone else's hurt.

And so with that in mind, here is a letter from Dr. Ramey to his daughter, not so very long ago.

~

Sarah,

I have been thinking about how you can end your book. I am sure you have thought of this already, but here goes.

I presume much of the beginning is about people's symptoms, the attitude of doctors toward their symptoms and individual stories.

What you might do is elucidate the theory that all the various syndromes are related—just different manifestations of the same underlying problem. Then describe what is known about the intestinal biome and how it is related, the immune system and how it is related, the endocrine system and how it is related, and describe where the research is going. Then describe what people can do now—resources in the city they live in.

Finally, you could describe the evolution of a by-the-numbers internist like me.

I now have a stable of eight patients with varieties of the mysterious illness. I put them on gluten-free diets, prescribe probiotics, keep them away from antibiotics, refer them to GI people like [Dr. Wonderful], acupuncturists, physical therapists, and sometimes supportive psychotherapists. I tell them they are not crazy, and they should soldier on. They love to have a doctor who understands their suffering and is working with them to help, even if I don't offer magic cures. You could emphasize that they all return for advice because I am the only physician they have seen who believes they have something wrong that is not psychiatric and I have some things to offer.

You could recommend that physicians as well as all the other professionals helping people with these problems educate themselves as to what is known intellectually about the syndrome and the resources in the community to help alleviate the distress.

Dad

~

When I got this, I wept.

You see, for so long my conversations with my father about the science of my illness were so contentious—me presenting my findings, my father presenting his extreme Doubt—that I eventually stopped talking about it with him. That was about six years ago.

I didn't know that in the interim my father had changed his mind.

I didn't know he had changed his medical practice.

I didn't know he had taken virtually all of my advice.

I didn't know he had stopped asking his more irritating patients if their left elbow hurt when they urinated.

I didn't know that my experience had changed *him*.

I had no idea that my dad, of all people, was now acting as a benevolent guide and friend to the WOMIs of Washington, D.C.

Dr. James N. Ramey:

Heroine.

And so let me be very clear.

If my father, *of all people*, can write this letter—if the great pooh-pooher himself can change his mind, change his medical practice, and change his relationship with his sick daughter—then my friends, hope and change are indeed possible, and they are on the way.

34

This brings us back to you, reader.

Our story does not end with a thrill, a diagnosis, an arrow up through the chink in Smaug's golden underbelly of armor. For all the high-flying rhetoric about the mythology, and calls to duty, and the saving of the interior, one initiate at a time, there is only one place to land, and that is with you.

And I know you may be very sick, you may be the partner of someone who is very sick, you may just be starting to get sick—or you may just be some poor soul who picked up a uro-vago-colo page-turner, and here we are.

And I know that these illnesses can feel like falling into an abyss of ugliness, where all control is lost, where health care providers are cruel, and where your life seems like it will forever be batted back and forth at the whim and mercy of your doctors and your body.

But I also know that when you eventually find yourself hitting the rock bottomest of rock bottoms, you do tend to realize that this is your one and only life—wild and precious, as Mary Oliver would say—and you have to claim it.

So as our time together draws to a close, whoever you are, here is what I wish for you.

If you have been crushed, and crushed, and then crushed again—
If you have been denied, and denied, and denied again—

If you have been erased, and disappeared, and pushed to the margins over and over and over again—

Remember:

The Book of the Dead is also the book of life.

Of all the things we have talked about at great length now, the only thing that actually matters is that you do only those things that bring *you* to life.

That is your glowing compass in the dark.

If changing your diet brings you to life, that is the right thing to do. If making a film about people like us brings you to life, that is the right thing to do. If coding a technology that will help people like us brings you to life, that is the right thing to do. If exercising a few minutes a day brings you to life, that is the right thing to do. If having more sex, if dancing more, if singing more, if laughing more brings you to life, then those are all the right and good things to do.

Your life is what matters.

Not ideology.
Not data.
Not gurus.
Not doctors.
Not me.

Your life, wild and precious.

And so in other words, my dear, patient, graceful, and elegant reader:

Instead of staying trapped in Hades forever:

May you be the girl who lived.

ACKNOWLEDGMENTS

I genuinely cannot believe we finished this book, major emphasis on the word "we."

If the thought has crossed your mind that it sounds hard to write a book while also participating in the Bowel Olympics, boy howdy are you right.

There is no way I would have been able to write this without the myriad types of support I received over the last fifteen years from friends, family, and my publishing team. So let's start at the beginning, and when we get to the end, stop.

First and foremost I want to thank my family—I really do not know where I would be without your love and support. Mom, you are a saint. Dad, you are my heroine. Jimmy, you are the jackpot of brothers. Meg, I love you so doggown much.

Anna Stein, my agent: I'm pretty sure this book would not exist without you. You are my friend, my cheerleader, my defender, my sometimes editor, and I will never be able to thank you for going so far above and beyond that I can barely see you anymore.

Kris Puopolo, my editor: The patience you have cultivated over the *ten years* it took for the book to go from proposal to print copy is difficult to fathom. I am deeply grateful for your unwavering support, belief, and guidance. Thank you.

Hugs, thanks, awards, and medals of honor also go to:

My friends! As someone who barely ever gets to see her friends because of this awful disease, I am profoundly grateful that despite it all you guys never let me go. Kelly McFarling and Megan Keely— the happiest I have been in two decades is singing in a room (any room) with you. Maeve O'Regan, Faith Rose, Cecily Upton, Liam Templeton, Katharine Smyth, Emily Weinstein, Cassidy Grattan, and Rajan Grewal—thank you for bearing witness, over and over and over again. Nick Stargu and Pete Lee, Wolf Larsen would be but a glimmer in my eye without you. And my dear Ethan Bullard and Colin Joyner: *Ask not For Womb the Bell Tolls* . . . this womb tolls for thee.

My village: Dru Ramey, Marvin Stender, Jessica Stender, Caitlin and Adam Schaffer, Daniela Michel, Fran Weiss, the Langevin clan, Ane Axford, Terese Taylor, Stacey Richter, Dan Coleman, Curtis McCrary, Carol Varney, Scott Pryor, Nathaniel Smith, Tucson song night, Zack Vieira, The Hotel Utah, HOPE/WILL, Courtney Hull, Alex Mitchell, Lottie Ryan, Briana Saussy, Danielle Ben-Veniste, Abby Cutler, Charlotte Band, Cat Price, Anne and David Kendall, Susan Clampitt and Jeremy Waletsky, Ken and Karen Christensen, Dana Weant and Melanie DeBoer, Tory Newmyer, Bobby Martin, Scott McCabe, Jonathan Kirchner and Emma Silvers, Micah DuBreuil, Jennifer Purrenhage, Lizzie Hooper, Rachel Riggs, and Ed Pierce. And of course the most gifted and powerful healer in this or any village, Mathilde.

My readers: Dr. Carole Horn, Dr. Nisha Chellam Vedamuthu, Dr. Linda Simoni-Wastila, Beth Raymer, Alisa Vitti, Nick Jaina, and Ed Yong.

My publishing house: Bette Alexander, Daniel Meyer, Daniel Novack, Todd Doughty, and especially Bill Thomas.

My publishing village: Ursula Doyle at Fleet, Jeanine Langenberg at Sebes & Bisseling Literary Agency, Elik Lettinga at Arbeiderspers, and Morgan Oppenheimer at ICM.

Every WOMI, MOMI, and HOMI who shared their dark and difficult story with me.

And finally, every doctor or nurse or practitioner who treated me with kindness and respect. A thousand blessings on your head.

RESOURCES

The Myalgic Encephalomyelitis Action Network: https://www
.meaction.net/
Open Medicine Foundation: https://www.omf.ngo/
Health Rising: www.healthrising.org
Stanford Medicine ME/CFS Initiative: http://med.stanford.edu/
chronicfatiguesyndrome.html
The Center for Complex Diseases: https://www.centerforcomplex
diseases.com/
Bateman Horne Center: http://batemanhornecenter.org/
Solve ME/CFS Initiative: https://solvecfs.org/
American ME and CFS Society: https://ammes.org/
International Lyme and Associated Diseases: https://www.ilads.org/
Lyme Action Network: http://www.lymeactionnetwork.org/
The American Chronic Pain Association: https://www.theacpa.org/
Black Health Matters: https://blackhealthmatters.com/
Invisible Disabilities Association: https://invisibledisabilities.org/
The Mighty: https://themighty.com/

FIND A FUNCTIONAL MEDICINE DOCTOR

https://www.ifm.org/find-a-practitioner/
http://www.functionalmedicinedoctors.com/
https://kresserinstitute.com/directory/

PODCASTS AND FILMS

The Doctor's Farmacy, with Mark Hyman
Revolution Health Radio, with Chris Kresser
FxMed, with Dr. Kara Fitzgerald
The Evolution of Medicine Podcast, with James Maskell
Unrest, Netflix
Fed Up, Netflix

FURTHER READING

Missing Microbes, Martin Blaser, MD
I Contain Multitudes, Ed Yong
For Her Own Good, Barbara Ehrenreich
The Empathy Exams, Leslie Jamison
Woman Code, Alisa Vitti
Food: What the Heck Do I Eat? Mark Hyman, MD
Total Recovery, Dr. Gary Kaplan
The Paleo Cure, Chris Kresser
The Autoimmune Solution, Dr. Amy Myers
The Wahls Protocol, Dr. Terry Wahls
The Hormone Cure, Dr. Sara Gottfried
The Athena Doctrine, John Gerzema, Michael D'Antonio
The Heroine's Journey, Maureen Murdock
Dancing in the Flames, Marion Woodman
Bluebird: Women and the New Psychology of Happiness, Ariel Gore

And because I cannot resist, here is Ramey's 10-Step, No-Fail, 100% Guaranteed Absolutely Works For Everyone, No Exceptions, Plan For Success:

1. Buy one cookbook by one of these functional medicine practitioners, and just stick to that. Simplify whenever possible.

2. Google "how to eat healthy on a budget" for good ideas, tips, tricks on how to save money.

3. Download a free or paid health coaching app to help keep you on track.

4. Seriously consider doing a supervised gut-healing program.

5. Seriously consider seeking out a functional medicine practitioner, or someone working in a similar model, especially if you have a difficult case. This is expensive, so if you're going to do it then plan to save up ahead of time, and only if you are prepared to do whatever testing and make whatever changes they ask of you. It's not worth it if you're hoping for a quick fix.

6. Join or start a Facebook group that supports you the way you need support. Some groups are solutions-focused, some groups are disease-specific, some groups are more for the airing of grievances—so pick what resonates with you the most, and try to make some friends who are like you. These may become some of your best friends, even if you've never met them in real life. Avoid the groups that submerge you in the suffering of others (unless you're into that, which is fine). I suggest looking for, or starting, one that encourages a sense of humor—I myself am always on the lookout for "gallows optimism."

7. Call your representatives in Congress and request that they stand up for funding ME/CFS and related disorders, and that they support initiatives such as the Healthy Food for All Americans Act. Do some research, look into what bills are on the table, and speak up. It takes five minutes, and a little bravery—but it really does matter.

8. Resist the Willy-Nillies! The wellness and medical industrial complexes are built to take your money, so be careful and deliberate with your plans.

9. Let how you feel be your ultimate guide—not how you look, not how much you weigh, not ideology, not what the newest study says. If what you're doing makes you feel better, you're doing it right. The science will eventually catch up to you.

10. Be absolutely sure to tweet chapter title puns to me @sarahmarieramey—just be aware that *Visit from the Poon Squad* has already been taken.

Goodbye, dear WOMI.
And good luck.

A NOTE ABOUT THE AUTHOR

Sarah Ramey is a writer and musician (known as Wolf Larsen) living in Washington, D.C. She graduated from Bowdoin College in 2003, received an MFA in creative nonfiction writing from Columbia in 2007, and worked on President Obama's 2008 campaign.